Learn to
Sleep
Well

CHRIS IDZIKOWSKI

CHARTWELL
BOOKS

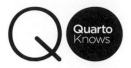

Inspiring | Educating | Creating | Entertaining

Brimming with creative inspiration, how-to projects, and useful information to enrich your everyday life, Quarto Knows is a favorite destination for those pursuing their interests and passions. Visit our site and dig deeper with our books into your area of interest: Quarto Creates, Quarto Cooks, Quarto Homes, Quarto Lives, Quarto Drives, Quarto Explores, Quarto Gifts, or Quarto Kids.

This edition published in 2016 by Chartwell Books, an imprint of The Quarto Group, 142 West 36th Street, 4th Floor, New York, NY 10018, USA
T (212) 779-4972 **F** (212) 779-6058 **www.QuartoKnows.com**

Conceived and produced by:
Watkins Media Ltd
359 Goswell Rd
London EC1V 7JL
United Kingdom

Chartwell Books titles are also available at discount for retail, wholesale, promotional, and bulk purchase. For details, contact the Special Sales Manager by email at specialsales@quarto.com or by mail at The Quarto Group, Attn: Special Sales Manager, 401 Second Avenue North, Suite 310, Minneapolis, MN 55401, USA.

ISBN-13: 978-0-7858-3463-2

10 9 8 7 6 5 4 3 2

Printed in China

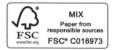

MIX
Paper from
responsible sources
FSC® C016973

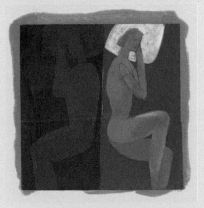

DEDICATION

For Tom and Molly and their extended family

Contents

Introduction   8

Sleep in Perspective   11
A Brief History of Sleep   12
What is Sleep?   14
Why Do We Sleep?   16
When Nature Sleeps   18
The Time for Sleep   20
Sleep at All Ages   22
The Sleep Record   24
Exercise 1: Logging Your Sleep
   Response   25

Patterns of Sleep   27
Sleep for All Seasons   28
The Body's Clock   30
Understanding Sleep Controls   32
The Rhythms of Sleep   34
A Journey in Time   36
Exercise 2: Finding Your
   Ninety-Minute Cycle   37
Crossing the Threshold   38
Into the Depths   40
Flutters in the Night   42
Sleep Bounces Back   44
Assessing Your Sleep Quality   46

The Sleep Environment   49
Blowing Hot and Cold   50
Peace and Quiet   52

Blissful Beds   54
Sleeping Partners   58
Exercise 3: The Gift of Touch   59
Co-sleeping with Children   60
Light and the Spectrum   64
Exercise 4: Finding Your Palette   65
Feng Shui in the Bedroom   66
Exercise 5: Clapping Out
   Trapped Qi   67
The Pa Kua Chart   70

The Sleeping Body   73
Sustenance for Sleep   74
Catching Sleep Thieves   78
Fitness for Sleep   82
Exercise 6: The Pre-sleep Stretch   83
The Indian Path   86
Exercise 7: Breathing Away Stress   87
The Chinese Traditions   88
Exercise 8: Acupressure for Sleep   91
Baths for Sleep   92
Exercise 9: Inhaling Calm   93
Soothing Touch   94
Exercise 10: Stroking Away
   Tension   95
Herbalism and Aromatherapy   96

A Mind for Sleep   101
Banishing Worries   102
Exercise 11: The Birds of Peace   103

Casting Off Anger   106
Exercise 12: Letting Go   107
The Power of Meditation   108
Exercise 13: A Candle-flame
    Meditation   109
Patterns of the Cosmos   112
Exercise 14: Creating Your Own
    Sleep Mandala   113
Visions of Sleep   114
The Power of Suggestion   116
Exercise 15: Enticing Yourself
    into Sleep   117
Sounds Asleep   118
Routines and Rituals   120
The Nature of Dreams   122
Exercise 16: How to Recall Your
    Dreams   125

Overcoming Sleep
    Problems   127
Defining and Tackling Insomnia   128
The Nighttime Marathon   132
The Terrors of Deep Sleep   134
The Terrors of Dreaming Sleep   136
Exercise 17: Spinning Out
    Nightmares   137
Sleep Paralysis and Narcolepsy   138
Stepping Out of Time   140
Exercise 18: Synchronizing
    Clocks   141

Crossing the World's Time Zones   142
Exercise 19: Dealing with Jetlag   143
Working in Shifts   144
Coping with Snoring and Apnea   146
Exercise 20: A Swansong for
    Snores   147
When Your Partner is the Problem   150
Conclusion   152

Bibliography   153
Index   154
Author's Acknowledgments   160

Introduction

Insomnia is one of the most common sleep complaints, chronically affecting between five and ten percent of Americans. As well as taking a toll on an individual's health, this debilitating disorder has far-reaching negative economic and social effects. It is perhaps surprising then how little patients and health practitioners alike know about sleep. And to makes matters worse, insomnia is only one aspect of poor sleep! So in order to learn about sleep improvement, we must first learn more about the mysterious, fascinating state that is sleep.

We all know how important good sleep is because at some time we experience sleeping badly. Like breathing, sleep is essential. However, while we cannot go without breathing, we can do without sleep for short periods, in the knowledge that our bodies will find a way to recoup our sleep deficit. Take, for example, bringing up children — one of nature's big sleep experiments. If parents, had not evolved to cope with the way that babies and small children interrupt our sleep, we would never have survived as a species!

Upon being born, we cannot walk — walking is a learned skill that requires a certain level of brain development. Sleep is similar. The brains of newborns are immature and all the infants' basic needs — food, comfort and sleep — follow a genetically-programmed blue print. It is only at around three months, when some parts of their brain have matured, that babies learn to sleep at particular times. And gradually, over the next two years, they begin to adopt a sleep pattern that is more in keeping with their culture

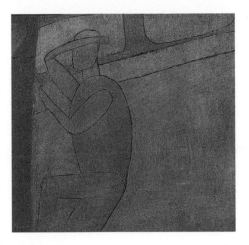

and, happily, more convenient for their parents. Sleep, then, is a part-learned behaviour.

As we grow older we inevitably experience stress, whether it is the tension that comes from our job, or the shock of a life changing event, such as bereavement. If we are lucky, any bad effect on our sleep will be only temporary, but if we are unlucky, the stress might cause us long-term sleep problems. If this has happened to you, take heart — you *can* re-learn how to sleep well, just as you originally learned your sleep pattern as a baby.

In *Learn to Sleep Well*, I provide an in-depth practical guide to teach you all you need to know to get a better night's sleep. Starting with an exploration of what sleep actually is, I delve deeper into the various bodily cycles and how these impact on our sleep, before looking at practical ways to improve our sleep environment. I then consider how we can adapt our lifestyle to help us to sleep better both physically and mentally, and I conclude with suggestions for dealing with specific sleep disorders. Good sleep is everybody's birthright. I hope that this book will help you to reclaim yours.

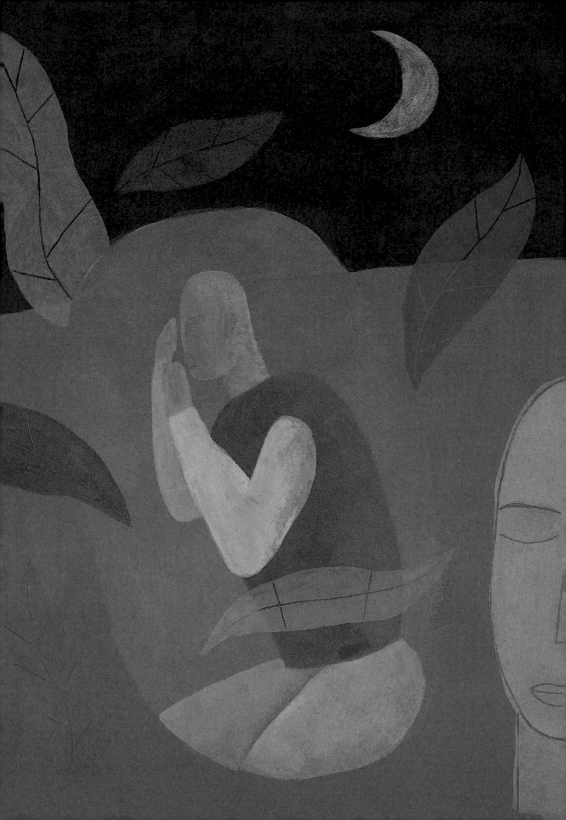

Sleep in Perspective

We spend approximately one third of our lives asleep. This is more time than we spend looking after our children; socializing with our friends; and more time even than working. Think how much effort we put into childcare, friendships and our jobs, and how little time we spend thinking about improving our sleep. We tend to take sleep for granted — we think of it as a revitalizing process that somehow should just "happen".

We are born with the gift of effortless sleep: when babies need to sleep they merely close their eyes and drift off. But by the time we reach adulthood, we have been taught to regulate our sleep habits according to the customs of our society. This learned behaviour supplants our ability to sleep naturally.

However, before we can take steps to improve our sleep, we need to understand it. In this chapter we explore what sleep is, and why and how we do it. We look at all the many ways in which sleep manifests itself — from the sleep-wake cycles of animals (and even plants) to the sleeping patterns of people across the world's cultures.

A Brief History of Sleep

All living things sleep. Some of them, such as humans, insects, plants, bacteria and many animals, switch in short-term cycles between rest and activity, while others undertake one prolonged stretch of inactivity — such as hibernating animals. However, despite the universality of sleep, and even despite the fact that sleep has been a source of fascination since ancient times, sleep research is still in its relative infancy.

When the ancient Greeks talked of Hypnos, they were referring to a mysterious god of sleep, who was said to live in a dark cave, and was the brother of Death and the son of Night. These dark associations suggest that the ancient Greeks were mistrustful of sleep — a state that they believed overpowered the brain against its will. Over time, medical men and philosophers tried to explain that state more scientifically. One of the more enduring suggestions was presented by Aristotle (384–322BCE) who believed that sleep was caused by the brain being "gassed" by the vapours of our food as the food decomposed in our stomach.

Notions of the brain being fumigated in the way that Aristotle had suggested or, alternatively, flooded with blood, abounded until the fifteenth and sixteenth centuries, when scientists discovered that such occurrences were physiologically impossible. The field of sleep research seemed at a loss — and by the eighteenth century the idea re-emerged that blood rising to the head put pressure on the brain, causing it to shut down temporarily.

After several other unsubstantiated theories, the breakthrough came in 1929 when German psychiatrist Hans Berger

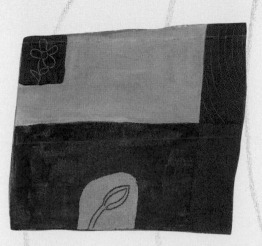

invented the EEG machine — the *electroencephalogram*. Berger claimed that this marvellous machine could measure different states of alertness by placing electrodes on a subject's scalp and recording the electrical activity of their brain (see pp.34–5).

Equipped with an EEG machine, in the 1950s the American psychologist Nathaniel Kleitman and his student Eugene Aserinsky made great leaps in the field of sleep research. Watching the sleep of infants, they noticed that for short periods the babies' eyes moved about rapidly behind the closed lids — and that each short period of eye movement corresponded with certain brain rhythms, read from the EEG. Thus REM (rapid eye movement) sleep was unveiled, shortly followed by further experiments and further readings from the EEG showing that there were four other, distinct stages of sleep (see pp.36–7). Most importantly, scientists came to realize that the brain is not passive or inactive during sleep as had been thought for hundreds of years — it chooses to sleep as a necessary part of our wellbeing.

The first positive steps in sleep science had been taken — only fifty years ago.

What is Sleep?

Sleep is far more than simple rest. We all do it and we all know from personal experience that its composition, depth and intensity, and its ability to refresh us, vary considerably. But how can we begin to define such a complex state?

We can start to characterize sleep by using our own powers of observation. Try watching someone as they sleep. They are probably lying inert in a peaceful, comfortable environment. They should be breathing steadily and quietly, and they may jerk and turn over from time to time. We may see their eyes moving beneath their eyelids, indicating that they are dreaming. The person is likely to be unresponsive to anything going on around them – although if we talk to them, they may give an incoherent reply. If we expose them to a strong enough stimulus, such as the sound of their baby crying or the ringing of an alarm clock, they will immediately awaken, although it might take a moment or two for them to become fully alert.

With these characteristics in mind, we might then look at how scientists have attempted to define sleep, drawing parallels with our observations where we can. For example, some researchers contrast sleep with wakefulness, describing the two as obverse sides of the same coin. If wakefulness is a time when we have complete self-awareness – when we can voluntarily do certain things such as eat, drink, think and work – sleep is the opposite. Just as we observed, in the sleep state we are generally physically inactive, except for minor unconscious movements, such as scratching. Special brain mechanisms dampen the amount of

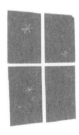

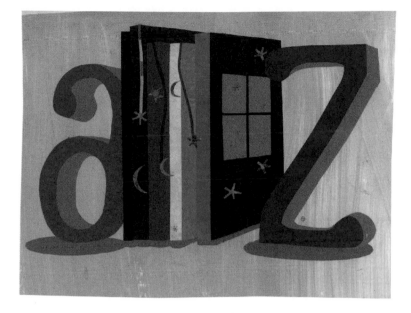

information that flows in from the senses, while other brain signals relax or even paralyze many of the body's main muscles. And although we are mentally active while we sleep — we have thoughts and see images in our dreams — our brain processes lack the structure and logic that they have when we are awake.

One final route to defining sleep is to break the state down into its physiological stages. On average, we clock up between six and nine hours sleep at night, during which time we go through four or five separate cycles, each lasting roughly ninety minutes. These cycles are interspersed with brief periods of wakefulness, which we do not remember. To further complicate matters, each sleep cycle has five stages (as elaborated by Kleitman's student Dement): drowsiness, light sleep, two stages of deep sleep, and REM sleep. A healthy adult's sleep comprises around 25 per cent deep sleep, 50 per cent light sleep and 25 per cent REM.

Why Do We Sleep?

Evolution, nature's own judge of the effectiveness of living things, would not require us to spend approximately a third of our lives asleep unless sleep offered some distinct physical or mental advantage. Before we begin the path toward sleep improvement, it is instructive to consider why we sleep at all.

We know that most sensory stimulation is shut out during sleep and our muscles are fully relaxed — some of them even temporarily paralyzed. We might say, then, that we sleep in order to force ourselves to rest. However, we would be wrong to interpret sleep simply as a means of energy conservation. The amount of energy saved during sleep is unremarkable: a person weighing 200 pounds (approximately 91 kg) burns off calories during sleep at a rate of 80 per hour. The same person sitting quietly uses up calories at a rate of 95 per hour — so the energy saving during eight hours sleep (compared with eight hours waking rest) is roughly equivalent to a glass of low-fat milk!

In a similar vein, some scientists have claimed that deep sleep is fundamental to repairing the daily wear and tear on the body, and that dreaming sleep restores the efficiency of the brain. We can see how we might arrive at this conclusion — it is an extension of the knowledge that animals with fast metabolisms sleep longer than those with slow ones. In other words, we sleep so that the body and mind are forced to stop and undertake internal maintenance work — in this way we are prevented from burning ourselves out. However, mounting evidence suggests that the body does not repair itself during deep sleep any more than during light sleep

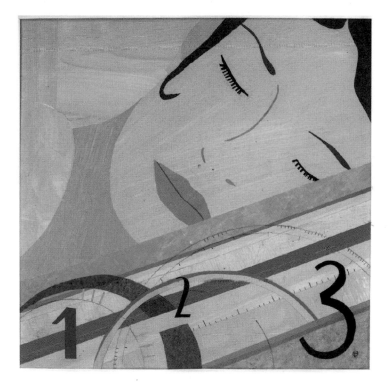

or wakeful rest, and that most of the brain is as active while we are dreaming as it is when we are awake (in fact, many psychologists believe that the activity of our brains during sleep – when we are in a period of dreaming sleep – is essential for our emotional and mental wellbeing; see pp.122–5).

So where does this leave us? We do not know for sure when sleep evolved, how it evolved, nor whether it evolved to have one or more functions. But the one thing of which we can be sure is that sleep is essential to survival – bacteria, plants, animals and humans all undergo periods of sleeping and, if it were not essential, evolution would have cast it aside from one or all of these living organisms many thousands of years ago.

When Nature Sleeps

So far we have learned that sleep is difficult to define and that the reasons for sleeping are elusive — even to the experts. Perhaps, then, we should step back and see if we can identify any keys to sleep that might provide a basis for sleep improvement.

The most obvious first step is to examine what we see in the world around us — beginning with nature. Think of the daily cycle of a daisy, say. The flower opens its petals with the dawn and closes them as the sun sets. Its nourishment (occurring through a process called *photosynthesis*, which converts the sun's rays into "food" — in the forms of oxygen and sugars — for the plant) is governed by the turn of each day from light to dark. We might therefore say that for the daisy (and thousands of other flowers and plants, of course) "work" (photosynthesis) occurs during the day, and "rest" occurs during the night — a pattern which seems very familiar to us. Making a direct comparison with human behaviour and the natural cycles of human life (see pp.28–9), we might conclude that taking note of the earthly cycle of light and dark is of fundamental importance to the quality of our sleep.

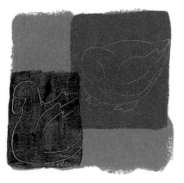

Apart from looking at plant life, scientists find it instructive to study the sleep behaviour of animals. Many experts believe that one of the keys to sleep lies embedded in the fact that different kinds of mammals (warm-blooded animals) have varying sleep times. For example, the brown bat is active for only four hours each day. Similarly, the North American opossum manages to clock up about eighteen hours' sleep each day. At the other end of the spectrum are the ruminating animals, such as cows and horses, which sleep as little as three or four hours in every 24. From this we glean that the bigger the animal and the slower the metabolism, the more sleep is needed.

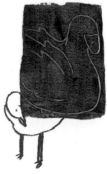

Animals also teach us that sleep is posture-specific — even crustacea adopt specific body positions and show changes in muscle movement when they rest.

By looking at the natural world, then, we learn of three key influences on human sleep: the natural cycles of light and dark; metabolism; and sleeping posture — which for humans means our environment as well as the position in which we sleep.

LEARNING FROM THE SMALLEST CREATURES

Swiss sleep researcher Irene Tobler has spent her entire career determining whether or not animals sleep and how their sleep is controlled. Among her more unusual discoveries is that cockroaches and goldfish sleep. But how can we tell? The way Tobler did it was to keep the goldfish and cockroaches moving about for long enough so that they had to have missed a period of sleep usual to their sleep cycle — and then (when she stopped pestering them!) she observed what happened. Having been deprived of sleep, the cockroaches and the goldfish became still for a protracted period of time — suggesting that the sleep deprivation had led to an increased need for them to rest. Tobler's discoveries have played an important part in leading sleep researchers to the conclusion that *all* animals — not just mammals — sleep.

The Time for Sleep

One of the most frequently asked questions about sleep is, What is a "normal" amount of sleep? If only it were that simple! Before we can begin to improve our sleep, we must understand one other fundamental principle about the way in which sleep works: namely that the amount we need varies from person to person. Sleep times depend partly on the way in which we are brought up and partly on our biological make-up. Furthermore, the unanswerable question ignores one important factor — we should not be asking simply, How much sleep do we need?, but also, When should we take it?

A siesta — an afternoon nap, usually taken during the hottest part of the day — is standard in many Mediterranean and tropical regions. Some might think that this is a luxury and that those who take a siesta benefit from "extra" sleep. In fact, things tend to balance out and, in cultures where the siesta is common, people usually stay up much later into the night than in non-siesta countries. Overall, siesta-takers may get around eight hours

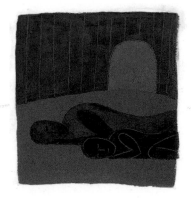

sleep (like most of the rest of us), broken into two unequal chunks (the first, a short burst of two or three hours; the second, a longer stretch of five or six).

Historically, the American Navajo people believed "A man lying down during daytime is a lazy man," but before the working day became a nine-to-five entity, all Western sleep patterns may have been more broken up. Some research has shown that the sleep of medieval peoples quite often occurred in three distinct parts — a siesta in the afternoon, an early evening nap, and another, longer sleep until dawn.

But is this arrangement of short bursts of sleep any better for us than one long, rambling sleep period? Certainly, most research suggests that we are not physically designed to sleep in a single block of time and that a nap during the day and a longer period of sleep during the night is exactly the way in which nature intended we should sleep. Indeed, "polyphasic" sleep (sleeping more than once in a 24-hour period) is the most common pattern for sleep throughout the animal kingdom with "monophasic" sleep (a single sleep period) lagging far behind.

ASSESSING YOUR SLEEP DURATION

There are no rules about how much sleep we need — we must listen to our bodies. Our society tends to dictate that we sleep in a "monophasic" pattern — a single period of sleep every 24 hours, which usually occurs during the night. Do not worry if your sleep time seems short (say around four or five hours) — some of us are built simply to need only a few hours. Similarly, while sleeping more than nine hours a day is rare, it is not cause for undue concern unless social factors (such as a job, or school) are affected. If you can answer yes to the following questions, you are probably achieving the right amount of sleep.

• Do you fall asleep quickly (in under 20 minutes)?
• Do you sleep right through without waking in the night?
• Do you wake up in the morning bright and alert?

Sleep at All Ages

*

Our sleep patterns vary throughout our lives. In general, we tend to need less sleep as we get older. An awareness of how, when and why the changes occur in our sleep can help us to separate our natural decline in sleep duration from sleep problems.

After we are born we sleep for a total of up to eighteen hours a day, experienced as bursts of sleep which are interspersed with periods of wakefulness, usually to feed. At three to four years of age, we have a total of around twelve hours sleep. We grow rapidly at this age, so we need mostly "deep" sleep (this is actually a scientifically-accredited stage of sleep and not simply a colloquial term for healthy, restorative sleep; see pp.40–41), which we experience mainly during the first half of the night.

During puberty we might assume that our sleeping patterns would be disrupted by the profound biological changes we experience. However, between twelve and eighteen, our sleep pattern (including the stages of sleep that we go through — from light, to deep, to dreaming and so on) changes very little. What does change is our awareness of our own social and sexual status. This increased awareness of self is thought to disrupt our sleep by intruding into our dreams, making them unpleasant, anxious, or erotic. Adolescent sleep is also influenced by peer and school pressures — especially during the week — resulting in sleep deprivation on school nights, and prodigious amounts of catching up at weekends!

During early adulthood, from the ages of eighteen to thirty, our sleep comes under new pressures as our lifestyle changes. While sleep

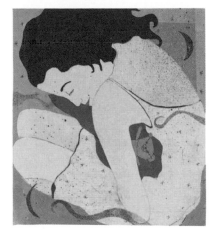

patterns are generally established by now and we might usually be getting the right amount of sleep, it is subject to the damaging influences of our changing circumstances – the pressures of a new regime of work and new financial responsibility, increased alcohol consumption, sharing a bed with someone else (perhaps someone who snores), newborn babies and so on. As we get older, sleep quality tends to worsen further – we tend to take less exercise and so gain weight, statistically we drink even more alcohol, and the years of anxiety that have built up in our minds and bodies release themselves in our dreams. Sleep during old age is mainly light and we suffer more frequent disruptions. Is it any wonder, then, that by the time we reach our 70s, we tend to compensate by napping during the day!

Taking an overview of a lifetime of sleep, what remains unclear is how many changes in sleep duration are irreversible. Having less deep sleep as we get older may be inevitable, but it does not necessarily mean that our sleep is less refreshing. Whatever age we are, we should always try to improve our sleep, so that we can enjoy each moment of wakefulness to the full.

The Sleep Record

The improvements we make to the quality of our sleep usually build up gradually, often so slowly that day-by-day changes are barely noticeable. One good way to monitor our progress is to keep a written record, so why not keep a sleep journal? This can be an invaluable tool for assessing what is going on in your sleep, before, during and after you start to tackle any sleep problems.

To help you get started, I have devised a "Sleeping Table", charting the progress of one night's sleep (a completed example is given below). It spans 12 hours from 9pm to 9am. In the evening note down anything you do, eat or drink between 9pm and the time when you try to go to sleep. Mark the moment you begin trying to sleep with a cross. Next morning, judge the point at which you actually fell asleep and mark it with a dot. If you got up in the night, draw an upward arrow and make a note of what you did (perhaps you had a glass of water or went to the bathroom). Draw a jagged line along the scale between the hours when you think you slept badly. For the period(s) when your sleep was peaceful, draw a solid line. Draw a dotted line for the period in the morning when you were semi-conscious, and an upward arrow to indicate when you got up. The exercise opposite tells you how to monitor your sleep over a 14-night period using this table as part of the process.

The Sleeping Table

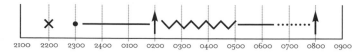

| 2100 | 2200 | 2300 | 2400 | 0100 | 0200 | 0300 | 0400 | 0500 | 0600 | 0700 | 0800 | 0900 |

Exercise 1

LOGGING YOUR SLEEP RESPONSE

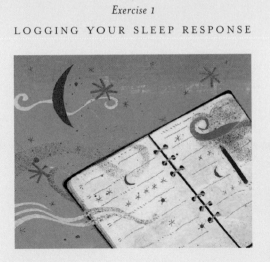

Follow the steps in this exercise for 14 consecutive days, without trying to improve your sleep. Two weeks should be long enough to give you an overview of how your sleep changes with variations in your lifestyle — after a night out with friends, a stressful day at work, days off, a difficult incident with your partner, and so on. Once you have your overview, try some of the improvement techniques in this book for one month, then repeat the experiment.

1. Prepare your journal. On a single sheet of paper, make a template page. Write "Day" and leave several lines' space where you can make notes about the events of your day. Beneath this, draw a Sleeping Table (described opposite). Leave space for any annotation to the table, then write the numerals one through 10 across the page. Note down that one represents "very drowsy" and 10 represents "very alert". Copy this template 14 times and write days and dates at the top of each page for the 14 days of your experiment.

2. Each evening complete the Day part of the journal and fill in the Sleeping Table. Next morning, as soon as you wake up, circle a number between one and 10 to indicate how drowsy/alert you felt on waking.

3. At the end of the two weeks, what can you learn about how occurrences in your daily life are reflected in the quality of your sleep? What steps can you take to neutralize the effects of the day on your nighttime rest?

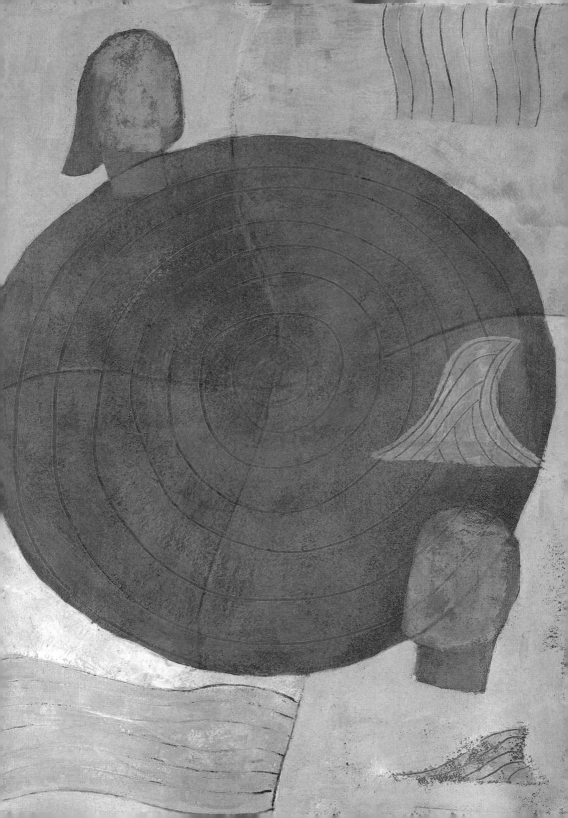

Patterns of Sleep

Since ancient times it has been known that sleep is composed of both dreamless and dreaming phases. With the discovery that the electrical activity of the brain can be used to identify five stages of sleep, new areas in sleep research have opened up over the past thirty years. This increased understanding has also led to the realization that the brain's biological clock has a profound influence on our sleep pattern and, in particular, on the amount of time that we spend asleep. Furthermore, it is now known that the brain has special control centres which cause sleep and wakefulness to switch on and off.

In this chapter we consider sleep in the light of this relatively new wisdom, gaining an insight into our nightly pattern, and learning how this knowledge might help us to improve our sleep. We conclude with a self-assessment — only once we have analyzed the quality of our sleep, as well as our lifestyle and our environment, can we really set about improving it on a permanent basis.

Sleep for All Seasons

It may seem an obvious point, but our body runs on cycles. We know this from simple experience – for example, the fact that we wake up in the morning and go to sleep at night, in a perpetual rhythm of action and inaction. However, we are also sensitive to several external cyclical patterns – in particular, the cycle of the seasons and the daily cycle of the sun. In order to fine-tune our sleeping patterns, we need to understand how these external, earthly cycles affect our inclination toward sleep itself. We start by looking at the impact the seasons have upon us.

The cycle of the seasons is a type of *infradian rhythm* (a cycle of more than 24 hours). The animals most affected by this are those that hibernate – with the onset of winter, they begin a prolonged period of dormancy, which enables them to survive the cold weather. Although we are not hibernating animals, we are also affected by the cycle of the seasons. During the night we produce the sleep-regulating hormone *melatonin*: the lack of light triggers the pineal gland in our brain to release it. This means that when the hours of darkness increase as winter creeps in, our melatonin production is stepped up, signalling to our body the seasonal change. The result is that we are naturally inclined to sleep for longer periods during winter (and for shorter periods during summer), and some researchers believe that this might even explain why many of us find it more difficult to get out of bed on winter mornings!

So, if we are having trouble sleeping, could we solve the problem by artificially increasing our melatonin levels? The hormone *is* available as a supplement in some countries. In the

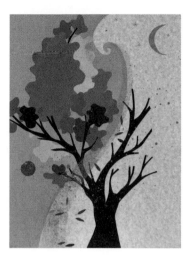

USA, melatonin is the only hormone that is not controlled by the US Food and Drug Administration; and it is taken widely there for its antioxidant and potentially life-prolonging properties. However, this is a powerful, regulatory hormone and, while it is clear that melatonin affects the biological clock, the jury is still out on whether it actually improves our ability to sleep. Either way, melatonin certainly should not be taken without adequate professional advice.

To help you to sleep well, it may be useful to become more aware of the effects that the seasons have on your body. Try to tune into their cycle – for example, watch not only how the leaves change colour in autumn, but also the myriad other little changes. Accept that you may feel especially sleepy during winter, and as far as is practical, allow your body to dictate your sleeping patterns. This will not mean that you will persistently oversleep during winter – you have an in-built *biological clock*, which partly regulates when you wake up. This, and the various other cycles which affect our sleep, are explained on the following pages.

The Body's Clock

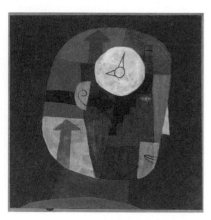

In order for us to be able to keep time with the cycle of the sun each day, we have an internal timekeeper, known as the "biological clock". In simple, neurological terms, this consists of a bundle of about 10,000 nerve cells, which are located deep in the brain near some of the main areas that control sleep and wakefulness. The nerve cells that make up the biological clock are also situated close to the optic nerves, which process information on the changing level of light perceived through our eyes.

Experiments have shown that the biological clock works on its own, roughly 24-hour cycle (in some people it is slightly longer and in others slightly shorter), and that the environment — in particular, changing temperature and fluctuations in light — serves to regulate the clock so that we all go to sleep and wake up on the same schedule, give or take a few hours. In other words, our environment sets the time, but the clock itself is preprogrammed and we would continue to have a roughly 24-hour cycle even if the sun never set and the temperature stayed at a constant level. Any 24-hour cycle is known as a *circadian rhythm*.

But what does this all mean for sleep improvement? Crucially, we need to determine whether our biological clock runs at a slightly slower or slightly faster pace than the cycle of the sun — that is, the 24-hour day. People who go to bed late and who consequently sleep through well into the morning have a biological clock running at a slightly slower pace than the 24-hour day — these people are often termed *owls*. Conversely, those who go to bed early but awaken early too have a biological clock running at a slightly faster pace — these people are termed *larks*. The box below helps to identify whether you are a lark or an owl — something you should bear in mind when you try to improve your sleep. For example, if you are an owl and you decide to go to bed an hour earlier than usual to try to get more sleep, you may well find that you spend that hour lying awake, worrying that you cannot sleep. Ideally, it would be more productive to allow your *biological clock* to dictate the *amount* of time that you spend asleep, while *you* take steps to improve the *quality* of that sleep.

ARE YOU A LARK OR AN OWL?

If you think about your own tendencies, you can probably guess whether you are a lark or an owl, but to confirm your analysis why not ask yourself the following questions?

- *Do you wake up bright and alert by 6am?*
- *Do you fall asleep quickly if you go to bed at 9pm?*
- *Do you find it hard to stay up until midnight?*

If you have answered yes to all three questions you are a lark.

- *Do you need to sleep until 11am to wake up bright and alert?*
- *Do you have trouble falling asleep before midnight?*
- *Do you fall asleep quickly if you go to bed at 1am?*

If you have answered yes to all three questions you are an owl.

Understanding Sleep Controls

In the twentieth century much progress was made in our understanding of how the human brain functions. During the First World War, there was a global epidemic of *encephalitis lethargica*, commonly known as "sleeping sickness". This debilitating disease, which killed approximately one million people, deeply affected sufferers' sleeping patterns, resulting in total lethargy (and ultimately death). However, amid the human tragedy a great scientific discovery was made — neurologists were able to ascertain that special "centres" exist in the brain to control sleep, and that these partly counter-balance equivalent centres, which maintain wakefulness.

Physiologically, our sleep and wakefulness controllers are located deep within our brain, a fact that indicates that their functions, while vitally important, are very primitive. There are three or four such areas in charge of sleep and approximately 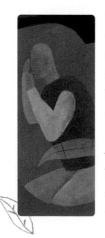 double that number for wakefulness, ensuring that, if one part of the brain becomes damaged, there are plenty of other areas that can take over its work. Some of the sleep centres are found near the controls for other important but basic functions, such as the regulation of body temperature, metabolism and appetite — and all these things have an impact on our ability to sleep well.

If a person's sleep centres are all active and their wakefulness areas are all inactive, they will experience a blissful state of sleep. However, if the person is disturbed — for example, by an uncomfortable bed, feeling too hot, experiencing pain or hearing a sudden noise —

their wakefulness areas will be alerted. These, in turn, will activate other parts of the brain that determine whether the stimulus warrants further action. If the disturbance is regarded as important, such as the sound of a baby crying or the smell of smoke from a fire, yet more parts of the brain will be switched on, bringing the sleeper closer to wakefulness. If the disturbance is regarded as insignificant, most of the brain will stay dormant and we will not actually achieve conscious wakefulness. And if we do wake up briefly, we will not necessarily remember it because an insufficient portion of our brain would have been activated for full consciousness to return. Whether or not we actually wake up, in the morning we will probably feel that we have had an unrefreshing night's sleep. From this we learn that our environment is a major contributor to the quality of our sleep – and a key to sleep improvement.

CONSCIOUSNESS AND WAKEFULNESS

*

In order to comprehend fully how sleep works, we must first understand the distinction between consciousness and wakefulness. The French philosopher René Descartes (1596–1650) famously wrote "I think, therefore I am," and thus described consciousness – we are conscious beings because we have an awareness of self and our environment. But what happens when we sleep? We know that consciousness does not disappear because we dream (even if we do not remember our dreams) – which might be considered "thinking" sleep. Wakefulness, then, is the part of consciousness that is "full", when we are wholly in control of our actions, and so on, and when we are aware of the world around us.

The Rhythms of Sleep

Before we move on to study the unique physiology of the human sleep-cycle, we need a basic knowledge of the behaviour of our brain, as we enter the various the stages of sleep.

The invention of the EEG in 1929 by Hans Berger led to major advances in sleep science by revealing that sleep is not a single, one-dimensional state, but rather a dynamic process during which the brain continues to respond to the environment and the internal functions of the body, while still overseeing the operation of sleep itself.

To get a better grasp of what goes on in our brain when we sleep, we need to look at the variations in the electrical activity of the brain at different times of the day, as well as of the night. When we are fully awake our brain activity is characterized by high-frequency, low-voltage brain waves called *beta waves*. The frequency of these waves varies according to the tasks that we are undertaking, as well as the amount of stress that we feel: the more active the task, or the more acute the stress, the higher the frequency of the beta waves. The waves gradually slow down as we become more tired toward the end of the day. Finally, when we relax with our eyes closed, beta waves turn into slower, relatively low-voltage *alpha waves*, which were discovered by Hans Berger. Then, as we become drowsy, the alpha waves become interspersed with even slower brain waves called *theta waves*. Drowsiness is a transition state — it lies between sleep and wakefulness. This is a time when we can easily return to wakefulness, but it is also a time when we might experience lifelike hallucinations, called *hypnagogic* dreams (see pp.38–9). However, if we are sleeping healthily, we

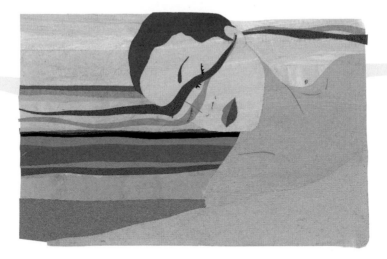

spend only a short period in Stage I sleep and we soon produce the fast, short bursts of waves (as shown on the EEG) called *sleep spindles* (because they look like the spindles used by hand spinners). These herald the first true sleep state – Stage 2, in which we fully lose our awareness of the outside world. These sleep spindles soon turn into *delta waves* which are very large and slow and characterize both Stage 3 and Stage 4 sleep. These stages represent the deepest levels of sleep.

There is a fifth stage of sleep – that discovered by Nathaniel Kleitman and his assistant Eugene Aserinsky in 1952, and termed REM (rapid eye movement; see pp.42–3). This stage is usually seen as distinct from the other four stages of sleep, because our brain is highly active and the brain waves displayed on an EEG reading resemble those shown during wakefulness. When we are asleep we will typically progress through stages I to 4, and return to Stage 2 before entering our first period of REM sleep. The nature of this sleep cycle is more fully explained on the following pages.

A Journey in Time

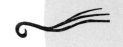

Sleep is not a linear phenomenon. When we are asleep, we do not progress continuously through the stages of sleep from light (stages 1 and 2) to deep (stages 3 and 4) to REM sleep. Instead, we make journeys back and forth (sometimes lingering longer or less in one place), up to five times a night. Each journey is a completed sleep cycle, which, in an adult, has been found to last approximately ninety minutes. (In babies the cycle takes approximately sixty minutes to complete.)

In people who are not suffering from health problems, and who are not taking any medication, the first and second cycles of sleep consist mainly of deep sleep (stages 3 and 4), with perhaps five to ten minutes spent in REM sleep in the first, and fifteen to twenty minutes in the second. As the night progresses, and we enter our third cycle, we spend most of the ninety minutes in light sleep (stages 1 and 2) and experience more REM sleep than in the previous two cycles. The fourth and fifth cycles are dominated by REM sleep, interspersed with light sleep.

So how might this knowledge of sleep cycles help us to improve our sleep? Interestingly, experiments have shown that the ninety-minute cycle may not be confined to sleep — it can also be found when we are awake (see opposite). Research has indicated that around every ninety minutes during wakefulness our concentration wanders, the nostril through which we breathe more air switches (our nostrils never share the work equally!) and our energy levels drop. By identifying these low-points in the brain's awake cycle and adjusting our bedtime to coincide with them, we may substantially improve our chances of falling asleep.

Exercise 2

FINDING YOUR NINETY-MINUTE CYCLE

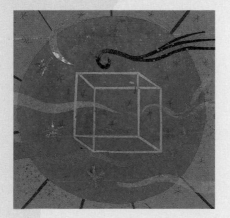

Using the following experiment, discover your own, waking ninety-minute cycle. Then, once you have established roughly the times when you are at your highest and lowest levels of alertness, make adjustments to your day. Try to undertake tasks which require most concentration when your cycle is at its peak, and go to bed at the low-point in your cycle, when you should find it easier to fall asleep. (As the experiment requires monitoring over a full day, it may be more convenient to conduct it at a weekend or on another day when you are not at work.)

1. Use the image above, or carefully trace over or redraw the cube part, to create a "portable" optical illusion. The cube, if looked at carefully for a period of time, will appear to switch the direction in which it faces — sometimes it will face downward as if toward the southeast and sometimes it will seem to point upward, toward the northwest.

2. Set an alarm to go off every 15 minutes throughout the day. Each time it rings, look at the cube. Time (by simple counting if you like) how long it takes for the cube to switch from one direction to the other.

3. After each occasion that you have looked at the cube, note down your "switch time". The rapidity with which the cube switches reaches a maximum every 90 minutes. The closer you are to the low-point in your cycle, the quicker *the cube will switch.*

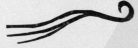

37

Crossing the Threshold

If we are healthy we should be able to fall sleep readily at the beginning of a ninety-minute cycle. Although identifying this cycle can be a great benefit in improving our sleep at night, other factors also affect our ability to go to asleep, which is actually a complicated process. To be able to fall asleep easily we have to rely upon our brain to switch off our wakefulness controls and at the same time to activate our sleep centres. In people who are not stressed, have not been overly active before they go to bed, and who are without sleep problems, this process is automatic. When we enter the first stage of sleep (Stage 1), if we are healthy, our muscles relax and our eyes roll beneath our lids. But if, for example, we are stressed, our wakefulness controls tell our brain that our muscles are not in the appropriate condition for sleep, and we have conflict between the sleep and wake controls, which will only be resolved once we start to relax.

Think back over the last week — how easily did you "drop off" each night? On some nights you probably fell asleep almost immediately, while at other times sleep might have been more elusive. In the first instance, there would have been a rapid progression from wakefulness to feeling drowsy and then into light sleep. When you were having difficulty falling asleep, however, you would have drifted in and out of consciousness and your final loss of awareness — the moment when you actually crossed the threshold into sleep — probably seemed to take for ever. At such times, when our brains appear to hover on the edge of awareness, many of us remember experiencing weird, dreamlike visions. These fragmentary images occur in a state known as

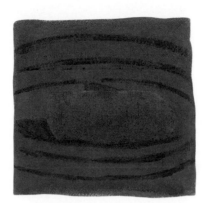

hypnagogia and are characteristic of Stage 1 sleep. What is more, the hallucinatory aspects of this sleep state can be so frightening that they have themselves been known to cause sleeplessness. (More rarely, similar experiences occur as we drift into wakefulness sleep — this experience is known as *hypnopompia*.) Although we cannot control hypnagogia or hypnopompia, it can help to know that they are a completely normal part of the falling-asleep process, and that any other apparently random experiences (for example, images of a loved one laughing, "hearing" the sounds of alarm bells ringing, and the common sensation of falling) are merely our imaginations playing tricks on us. Perhaps — more romantically — we might like to think of the visions as temptations from the dreamworld, inviting us to sleep.

When we finally succeed in falling asleep (and assuming that we average eight hours' sleep per night), we spend roughly fifty per cent of this time in light sleep. However, this is mostly made up of Stage 2 sleep. Our periodic return to Stage 1 is usually only fleeting and is characterized by a change in sleeping position — it is rarely significant enough for us to recollect having drifted into near-wakefulness.

Into the Depths

When we are healthy in body and mind, and our sleep is healthy too, we usually move out of Stage 2 and into Stage 3 sleep within ten to fifteen minutes of trying to drift off. However, we normally spend very little time in Stage 3, and as soon as our brain waves have slowed down to comprise more than fifty per cent delta waves (high-voltage waves, oscillating at a rate of around one wave per second), we reach Stage 4 sleep — the deepest level of all. The first third of our sleep is mostly made up of Stage 4 sleep. The duration of each period of deep sleep becomes shorter as the night wears on.

The importance of Stage 4 sleep for our overall wellbeing is reflected in the fact that it takes precedence over the other stages. Experiments have shown that if we are deprived of sleep for one night we usually make up *almost all* the lost deep sleep on the following night (mostly at the expense of lighter sleep). Even if we are made to go longer without sleep — say, for two or more nights — practically the entire deep-sleep debt is recouped over the course of our next two or more nights' sleep.

Similarly, when the sleep patterns of constitutionally short-sleepers (people who have only between four and five hours' sleep every night but feel perfectly well) are compared with constitutionally long-sleepers (those who need around nine or more hours' sleep to feel well), it is apparent that both types spend approximately the same amount of time in deep sleep — around two hours in total per night.

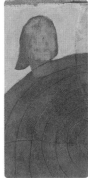

If deep sleep, then, is the most essential stage of sleep and our bodies are programmed to ensure that we always eventually make up any deficit (see pp.44–5), we may wonder why we might still feel unrefreshed and tired on any given morning. The answer to this question is that although deep sleep is the most important for our actual physical wellbeing (scientists believe that crucial maintenance and restoration work is done to the body during deep sleep; see box below), our waking sense of wellbeing arises from learned feelings of wellness, which usually require us to have had complete, uninterrupted sleep, comprising all sleep stages. In particular, we know that REM or dreaming sleep has a profound role to play in our overall physical and, especially, our emotional wellbeing. We consider this sleep stage next.

THE RESTORATIVE POWER OF DEEP SLEEP

When someone wakes us up and we feel temporarily disorientated, we often protest that we were "deeply asleep". However, it is unlikely that we were in what is scientifically classified as deep sleep (stage 3 or 4 sleep) as it is extremely difficult to be woken up during this part of the sleep cycle. Research has shown that this could be because deep sleep offers a guaranteed period during which the growth hormone can stimulate development in children and repair the blood cells and body tissue in adults. Recent evidence suggests that repairs to the brain as well as the body are carried out in this stage of sleep. If we are successfully roused from deep sleep, we may act as if intoxicated – behaviour known as "sleep drunkenness".

Flutters in the Night

If we look at the EEG reading of a person in REM sleep (rapid eye movement — so called because during this period of sleep our eyes dart quickly back and forth beneath our closed lids), the trace made by the EEG machine will resemble that of someone who is awake — in other words, the activity of our brain during REM is akin to that of wakefulness. Despite this brain activity and the movement of our eyes at this time, the muscles in almost all the other parts of our body (the exceptions being those that are essential to sustain life) become paralyzed. Because of the contrast between the activity of the brain and eyes and the paralysis of the muscles, REM sleep was once known as *paradoxical sleep*.

REM – SLEEP'S HARMONIZER

According to Hindu tradition there are three levels of consciousness — waking, dreamless sleep and dreamful sleep. The tradition goes on to say that, in order to live in balance and harmony, we must optimize our experience of all three. Although we might think that dreaming sleep is unimportant — a frivolous mode of expression for an overactive imagination — by depriving subjects of REM sleep, scientists have been able to *prove* that if we do not dream we become irritable, vague and easily fatigued, and we display a poor ability to remember things. This discovery reinforces the knowledge that recouping REM sleep is a priority over recouping light sleep in order to ensure our overall wellbeing.

But why are our muscles paralyzed during REM sleep? The logical explanation seems to be that this is a safety precaution to prevent us from acting out our dreams, most of which occur during REM. Centres in the brain actively block the output from the centres that normally stimulate movement. This might also explain the common dream experiences of being unable to run or incapable of screaming — perhaps such dream sensations are the mind's interpretation of the body's physical paralysis.

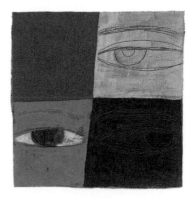

A healthy, young adult has approximately two hours of REM sleep per night, which occurs mainly in the second half of our sleep period. The "depth" of REM sleep lies somewhere between light and deep sleep. If we are roused during the REM phase of our sleep cycle we tend to be coherent and able to report the dream that has just been interrupted. However, our memory of dreams usually fades quickly (probably because long-term memory storage takes place during REM and normal, waking memory processes are not themselves yet awake!). This means that the longer the interval is between the end of REM sleep and the time we wake up, the less likely it is that we will be able to recall our dreams.

As with deep sleep, if we are deprived of the REM stage, our body will try to make up the deficit by prolonging the time we spend in REM on subsequent nights. Interestingly, going without sleep for a protracted period can even cause REM brain activity (and dreaming) to occur when we are awake, suggesting that dreams may be vital for our psychological wellbeing. By exploring the nature of dreams we can learn more about the role they have to play in improving our overall sleep (see pp.122–5).

Sleep Bounces Back

Now that we know about the cycles and stages of sleep, we are ready to set about assessing the quality of the sleep that we do obtain. However, just before we move on, there is one important thing to remember — sleep bounces back! There are times when our regular, 24-hour sleep–wake cycle is disrupted — sometimes for extended periods of time. For example, this might happen if we need to provide long-term care for someone who is ill, if we have a baby or if we work in an industry that sporadically requires us to work at night. Although we may feel nervous about the dangers of sleep debt, we should always keep in mind that the body has ways of ensuring that we get all the sleep we need:

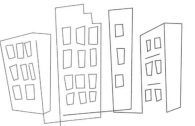

we already know that deep and REM sleep are made up at the earliest opportunity. (Constitutionally short-sleepers compensate for the short duration by foregoing most light sleep, gaining instead only two hours of deep sleep and two hours of REM.)

However, it would barely be sleep science if it were entirely that simple! There is, of course, a downside to our body's remarkable and innate ability to claim back the sleep debt. If we are sleep-deprived, "unintentional" sleep (the kind that occurs when we should be awake) invariably descends upon us when we are doing something monotonous and boring. One of the most obvious examples is the drowsy, luring kind of sleep that threatens to overwhelm us when we make a long and tedious journey on a highway, having started out feeling tired anyway. (Research has shown that doctors and nurses are more likely to be

involved in road traffic accidents when they have
worked an extended shift.)

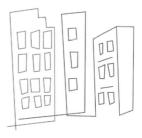

As a species we would not have survived this long
if conditions that constantly interrupt our sleep,
such as looking after children, could have a devas-
tating effect on us. Sleep has its own band-aid that
any of us can take advantage of at any time — the
nap. (Remember though, if you nap: it can take up to twenty
minutes to awaken fully and your "performance efficiency" — the
optimum level of alertness — lags behind your revitalized energy;
and napping when we are not suffering considerable sleep deprivation can upset the normal working of your biological clock.)

The most important point here is: if you think you are losing
sleep — don't panic! Your body will make up any sleep debt and
once you have been through this book and optimized the conditions for sleep, there will be every reason for sleep to be your
faithful nighttime companion.

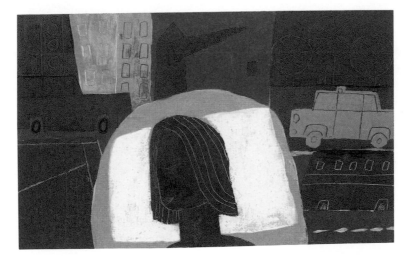

Assessing Your Sleep Quality

We should not begin to think about improving our sleep without first establishing what is wrong with it and what aspects of our lifestyle affect it. Only one fifth of the world's population enjoys perfectly healthy, restorative sleep. At best, the rest of us find ourselves falling asleep, say, as we read a book, and at worst suffer from a sleep disorder, such as insomnia or sleep apnea.

Begin by assessing your energy levels. Do you wake up feeling groggy or heavy-headed? Do you feel sleepy (or worse, fall asleep) at inappropriate times, such as during a meeting at work, listening to a lecture on the radio, or even watching your favourite television show, a good play or an exciting movie? Does your energy slump significantly after lunch? Do you wake up in the night? When you feel sleepy during the day, does the impulse feel all-consuming and almost uncontrollable? If you answered yes to most or all of these questions, your sleep quality is not as good as it could be! But do not worry — help is at hand!

We already know that there are three main conditions that affect sleep: mental and physical health and the sleeping environment. Listed opposite are a series of statements to help you assess your lifestyle and overall wellbeing. Note down whether they are true or false when applied to your circumstances. *Any* true statements can impair your ability to sleep properly, and you should prioritize these issues when beginning a sleep-improvement program. Then, look at all the other areas and take steps to deal with those too. Monitor your progress in a journal by noting when you go to bed, how long it takes to fall asleep, how long and how well you sleep, and how you feel when you get up.

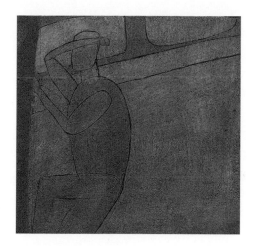

ASSESSING YOUR MENTAL WELLBEING
- I am quick to lose my temper or become irritable
- I laugh less than I used to
- I find it hard to concentrate
- I often feel on edge and tense
- I often feel sad or lonely

ASSESSING YOUR PHYSICAL WELLBEING
- I exercise less than twice a week (a brisk walk of about 20 minutes counts as the smallest unit of exercise)
- I often feel lethargic or sluggish
- I drink more than the recommended number of alcohol units per week (ask your doctor for the exact figure)
- I sometimes find it difficult to breathe
- I often suffer from muscular pain

ASSESSING YOUR SLEEPING ENVIRONMENT
- My mattress is lumpy/more than ten years old
- My bedroom is too cold/hot and stuffy
- I have a computer/television in my bedroom
- I have noisy neighbours/live on a busy and noisy street

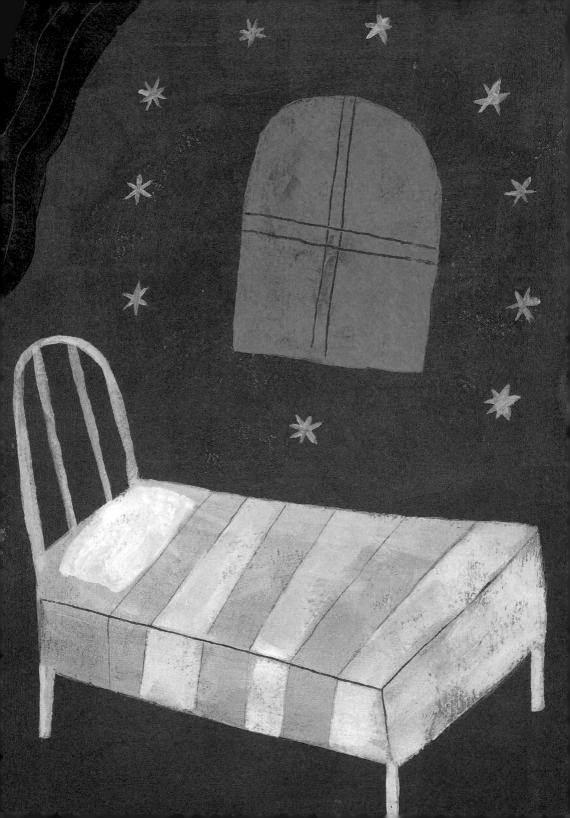

The Sleep Environment

The Victorian novelist Charles Dickens believed that it was important for us to sleep with our heads pointing north-ward. So strong was his view that he carried a compass around with him to ensure that no matter where he slept, he was always oriented in the right direction! Certainly, the precise location of our bed within our bedroom, as well as the comfort of the mattress on which we sleep and the variations of light in the room, can have a profound effect upon our quality of rest.

In this chapter we look at all these factors, as well as how to get the best from many common nighttime situations. We consider how to keep ourselves at a comfortable temperature throughout the night; we explore the effects of noise on our sleeping patterns; we learn how to obtain the most rest while sleeping with another adult in our bed and how to co-sleep peacefully with small children. We conclude with a lesson in the Chinese art of Feng Shui, with its focus on placement therapy — time-honoured techniques specific to the bedroom that can help us to balance the *qi* (energy) in our sleeping envi-ronment and ensure that we achieve optimum rest.

Blowing Hot and Cold

The temperature of our sleeping environment, both within our bedroom and in the bed itself, can have a profound effect on the quality of our sleep. For example, extremes of cold or heat cause shivering or excessive perspiring, which are likely to either disturb sleep or prevent it altogether. So what is the ideal room temperature for good sleep?

Dictating the optimal level can be difficult, as our ability to cope with temperature varies from person to person. The important thing is to find a level that feels right for you. As a guide, however, research has shown that 62°F (16°C) is generally conducive to restful sleep, while temperatures above 71°F (24°C) are more likely to cause restlessness. Childcare experts recommend that a baby's room is kept on a reasonably even level at 65°F (18°C).

However, keeping our environment at a constant temperature throughout the night does not guarantee good sleep. Our own body temperature changes according to our biological clock, normally reaching its warmest during the early evening, before dropping again in preparation for the night and reaching its coolest at around 4am. Ideally, then, the temperature of our room should follow this cycle, so that in winter we set our heating to go off in the evening and to come on again in the early morning. And in summer we should have the air-conditioning on during the evening *and* through the night, and let it go off as our waking time approaches. If this is not practicable, we can try other measures to control the temperature of our sleeping environment, such as keeping the drapes (which should be lined, preferably with white material to reflect the sunlight) drawn shut during hot summer days, as well as using heavier drapes in the winter to prevent the warmth of the central heating from escaping outside.

While Marilyn Monroe apparently slept wearing only a splash of Chanel No.5, most of us prefer to dress in at least a thin garment for bed. Whether you wear a nightshirt or a negligée, the composition of the fabric affects the exchange of heat and moisture between your body, your clothing and the layers of your bedding. For maximum sleep comfort you should always choose loose-fitting nightwear made from natural fabric such as cotton, wool or silk — and save lacy, frilly outfits for special occasions!

DEALING WITH HUMIDITY

*

Although we may not be aware of it, the amount of moisture in the air in our sleeping atmosphere is an important consideration for sleep quality. Bedroom air that is too dry can irritate the bronchial passages, causing us to awaken coughing. This can be rectified with humidifiers or simply by leaving a bowl of water in the room overnight. Conversely, excessive humidity, making us uncomfortably warm or damp, can raise our stress levels. If this is a problem, it is important to use bed linen made from natural fabrics which absorb perspiration and allow the skin to breathe.

If you are in a humid climate, you may be tempted to sleep without any clothes or covers. However, in humid conditions perspiration is slow to evaporate; if our body stays damp we may catch a chill. A better solution is to wear a thin, cotton garment or cover yourself with a cotton sheet, and use a ceiling fan to circulate air.

Peace and Quiet

Most people think they need complete peace and quiet in order to fall asleep, but as absolutely peaceful conditions rarely exist, this is an erroneous assumption. If you do manage to find a haven of tranquillity you might actually find it difficult to sleep, as many of us are used to going to sleep with at least some noise going on in the background. While intrusive sound, such as the electronic wailing of a car alarm, is likely to wake us up, pleasant noise can actually promote sleep. With a little experimentation we can discover which noises can help us to nod off (what is useful for some can be annoying for others), but to do this it is helpful first to understand how we perceive sound while we are sleeping.

Our ears convert noise into nervous impulses that are then recognized by the brain. Normally, perception is regarded as a conscious, waking phenomenon, but many of the systems that permit sounds to be experienced remain active during sleep and their performance may be observed using EEG machines. Our auditory systems certainly operate in light and dreaming sleep. If you call someone's name when they are in these sleep states, they will either start to wake up — you can actually see the brain waves change as the sound is interpreted — or your voice will be incorporated into the sleeper's dream.

During deep sleep (stages 3 and 4), even the higher processing centres are switched off, which is why it is so difficult to wake someone up in this part of their sleep cycle. But while the brain actively stifles the neural pathways that conduct sound when we sleep deeply, it does not turn them off completely, and some acoustic information filters through. The brain then interprets the messages and, if it recognizes that there is an emotional connection, wakes us accordingly. This is why mothers whose babies sleep in the same room wake up in response to the infant's smallest murmurs, whereas the same women may be able to sleep undisturbed through their partner's much louder snoring.

What noises, then, can be beneficial to sleep? Most experimental work to date has used either white noise (high-frequency noise that sounds like hissing), which with some imagination can resemble the ocean, or the real sounds of the sea, which are thought to have a calming effect and aid sleep. Next time you visit the seaside, try sitting on the beach and closing your eyes while you listen to the rhythm of the waves breaking on the shore – you will find yourself relaxing and, if you stay a while, you may even drift off to sleep. Both intensive care and premature baby units have investigated whether such ocean sounds can help to mask the general hubbub of hospital departments and promote sleep. The results so far have been encouraging, with patients showing significant improvements in sleep depth, as well as fewer awakenings and an ability to return to sleep faster.

Conversely, when sleeping, we should avoid background noise that can disturb us enough to affect our brainwaves without being intrusive enough to wake us up, as this can have a bad effect on our sleep cycles. For example, recent experiments show that the combination of vibration and noise caused by heavy road traffic going past participants' houses affected their sleep adversely by reducing their REM sleep. The people who took part in this experiment reported that they had noticed a decline in the quality of their sleep, a fact borne out objectively when their performance levels in subsequent mental tests suffered.

Blissful Beds

If upon waking we have aches and pains that dissipate after two or three hours, the chances are that our bed is to blame. Research has shown that simply by changing from an uncomfortable bed to a comfortable one, an individual will stir less and sleep longer. Our bed, or other sleeping surface, then, has a crucial part to play in the quality of our sleep. And, while lifestyle changes for sleep improvement may seem daunting or slow, buying a new bed is quick and easy, as well as effective.

There is no such thing as a standard sleeping surface – people around the world sleep on many different types, including futons, hammocks or water beds (all covered on p.57). But in the West, most people sleep on a mattress on a bed.

Research has shown that the material in most mattresses will have deteriorated by up to 75 per cent after ten years of use. Sleepers contribute to this decline by perspiring (we lose almost a half-pint or a quarter of a litre of fluid per night) and shedding about a pound (approximately half a kilogram) of skin per year. You should aim to replace your mattress every decade.

So what are the most important factors to consider when acquiring a new bed? The basic things you need to look at are the width and length, and the type of base and mattress. A bed should be as wide as possible – even if you sleep alone (of course, if you sleep with a partner you are less likely to be disturbed in a wider bed by his or her nighttime movements). It should also be four to six inches (10–15cm) longer than the tallest person intending to sleep in it, as you increase in height by approximately one inch (2.5cm) during sleep, owing to the rehydration of your spinal disks. If you are very tall, you can have a bed tailored to your own specifications by one of the manufacturers who offer custom-made beds. The base of your bed (no matter how tall you are) will depend upon the degree of firmness that you require in a bed, but the options range from divans with sprung interiors (made from materials similar to those used in mattresses), to hard, flat, metal bars or wooden slats.

HOW TO BUY THE RIGHT BED

Take your time when choosing a new bed, and do not be pressurized by over-enthusiastic salespeople. Always look for comfort and the level of support that is right for you. When trying out new beds in the store, take off your shoes, and lie on the bed in your usual sleeping position for at least 10 minutes.

FOR THOSE WITH BACK PROBLEMS
Orthopedic (which often just means firm) mattresses are included in most ranges. If you are not sure whether a bed is suitable, it is best to seek guidance from your doctor or other medical expert.

FOR THE ELDERLY OR PEOPLE WITH DISABILITIES
Consider the height of the bed and how easy it is to get in and out. Also assess whether you would be able to turn the mattress easily. Adjustable beds are worth considering if you need to sleep with your back in a raised position.

FOR THOSE WITH ALLERGIES OR ASTHMA
Most mattresses will attract dust mites, so choose one that is easy to turn and clean. Ask what fillers have been used in case you are allergic to any of them.

However, perhaps the most important component of a bed is the mattress, which should always be matched to fit the base of the bed perfectly. Mattresses consist of three main parts: the support, which usually comprises either springs or foam; the fillings; and the cover, which is also known as the "ticking". Mattresses should feel comfortable and should mould to the shape of your body; generally, the higher the number of springs used, the better the support. To check whether your mattress offers appropriate support (you can also do this when you go to buy a new mattress), lie on your back and try sliding the flat of your hand under the small of your back. If the mattress is too soft, you will have trouble getting your hand underneath; if it is

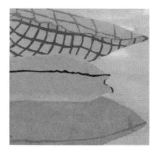

too hard, your hand will be able to move about freely as there will be a gap between the mattress and your spine. You will know when you find the ideal support, as your hand will fit snugly under the small of your back and the mattress will allow your spine to rest in its natural "S" shape.

Once you have ensured that your body is properly supported, you must pay the same attention to your head. There are pillows offering various levels of support, depending on your preferred sleeping position. In general, if you sleep on your back or side, you can use a firmer pillow than if you lie on your stomach. While feather pillows mould better to the shape of your head than other types, they are also expensive and can cause allergic reactions, including asthma and rhinitis. Good-quality pillows made from foam or synthetic fibres are now widely available. They are also practical, as they can be washed by machine. Babies should not have pillows until they are at least one year old, because of the danger of suffocation.

The next thing to consider after you have chosen your bed, mattress and pillows, is your bedding, which can affect not only your comfort levels, but also your body temperature (see pp.50–51). Today, quilts or duvets, which fashion themselves closely to the body, are very popular in the West. However, they are not suitable for babies under one year of age, who should instead sleep between cotton sheets, covered with cellular blankets. Some adults also still prefer traditional sheets and blankets, as layers can easily be added or taken off according to preference. As with beds, mattresses and pillows, the natural materials of cotton and wool as well as natural fillings are the most healthy, unless you develop an allergic reaction to them.

SPECIAL SLEEP SURFACES

WATER BEDS
These automatically provide the right support, distribute weight evenly and eliminate pressure points. Hygienic and non-allergenic, they consist of a water-filled vinyl mattress with soft foam or firm wooden sides.

FUTONS
Traditional in Japan, futons are usually made of layers of cotton wadding. The firm, unsprung sleeping surface moulds itself well to the body. They need good ventilation and frequent shaking to stop them from becoming hard.

HAMMOCKS
Cotton hammocks are portable, hygienic and ideal for hot climates, because they allow air to circulate around the surface of the body. And perhaps best of all, if you find yourself lying awake, you can gently rock yourself off to sleep.

Sleeping Partners

Most of us spend our childhood and adolescence sleeping alone in our own bed, often in our own room. It is only usually when we marry or form a long-term relationship with a partner that we have to adapt to sharing a bed. While sleeping with someone else can be a disruptive experience, there is evidence to suggest that it can also improve the quality of our sleep.

Research since the 1930s consistently shows that sleepers move between ten and twelve times per hour and that more than half of these movements involve major changes in position. So does all the tossing and turning disturb our partner's sleep? It is true that people who habitually sleep together usually move around less when their "other half" is absent (suggesting there are fewer disturbances), but studies have also shown that young couples tend to synchronize their movements while asleep. Interestingly, older partners who have spent longer together move less in harmony, which might be one of the reasons why we experience more sleep disruptions as we get older.

Partners can bring other advantages to satisfying sleep. A skilful massage produces a profound feeling of mental relaxation as well as a release of physical tension. This can also lead to an exploration of sensual pleasures with our partner and help us to maintain emotional intimacy with them. The warmth, comfort and sense of wellbeing that result from massage all encourage an excellent night's sleep. The pre-sleep massage opposite will encourage you both to relax. Or you could meditate together (see pp.108–11) before going to bed.

Exercise 3

THE GIFT OF TOUCH

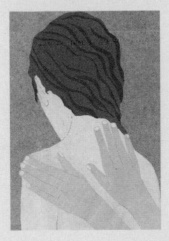

Mutual massage is a two-way exchange of touch and response between a giver and a receiver. It is the perfect way to harmonize your energies and reinforce your relationship so that you sleep more in tandem and reduce the amount of disruptive movements that you each make during the night. Try the following simple shoulder massage with your partner before you go to bed, taking turns in the active and passive roles.

1. Create a tranquil atmosphere in a peaceful room in the house (but not the bedroom) by dimming the lights and playing some gentle music. Light a scented candle whose fragrance reminds you of happy, lazy times spent together.

2. Place a towel on the floor and ask your partner to lie there on their stomach, head turned to one side. Place your thumbs between their shoulder blades on either side of the spine, your fingers resting on their shoulders.

3. Rotate your thumbs outward in small, rhythmic, circling movements, working a short way down your partner's spine and then out toward their shoulders.

4. With your partner's head turned to the right, squeeze the muscles of the left shoulder between your fingers and thumbs; gently knead the tension away. Turn their head to the left and repeat on the right shoulder. Now swap roles.

Co-sleeping with Children

Sleeping arrangements for babies and children vary considerably across cultures and ethnic groups. Climate, house-size, number of children, and the significance that parents attach to privacy all have an impact on where offspring sleep. In the West

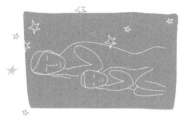

it is accepted practice for babies to sleep in a cot (and for older children to have their own beds), but in other parts of the world it is usual for children, especially babies, to co-sleep with their mother, or sometimes both parents. Putting infants to sleep alone is a relatively recent phenomenon, and as yet no conclusive studies have been conducted to assess the effect on children. However, more and more Americans and Europeans are discovering that sharing a bed with their baby, however unorthodox it may at first seem, is a perfectly practical step that can result in improved sleep for all the family.

Until the eighteenth century it was normal practice for Western families, regardless of means or status, to share a bed. It is only since the eighteenth century, when the medical profession first started to give advice on childcare, that mothers have been instructed to teach babies and children to sleep separately, in their own beds. This view was advocated by the famous American pediatrician Dr Benjamin Spock in his bestselling *Baby and Child Care*, first published in 1946, which even today influences the upbringing of millions of American children. However, not all families have adopted these recommendations. For example, research has shown that African-Americans frequently co-sleep with their children, and Appalachian families also ignore Dr Spock's advice, with about two-thirds of babies sleeping in their parents' bed or next to it. Many white American parents allow their children to co-sleep with them for part of the night when the youngsters need extra comfort because they are sick. Parents in Japan and Italy also have a long tradition of sharing a bed with their infants. Perhaps cultural variations in sleeping habits reflect fundamental differences in attitudes to independence — while the majority of American parents believe that children should become independent as soon as possible, African-American, Appalachian, Japanese and Italian families encourage more interdependent family links throughout life.

There are advantages in co-sleeping for both children (whether newborn or older) and parents. From the toddler's

NATURAL SLEEP REMEDIES FOR BABIES

If swaddling, rocking or lullabies have failed to coax your baby to sleep, you could try giving him or her a herbal tea instead. (All of the following are safe for children to drink, but it is always advisable to consult a herbalist before giving any remedy to a child.)

Camomile is one of the most popular and well-known herbal remedies, making a calming and soporific tea — give it to your baby tepid from a bottle or cup (see p.79 for full details on making herbal teas). You could sweeten it with a little honey for older babies (honey should not be given to a child under one year). *Dill* has also been used for centuries to tempt babies into sleep — the name actually derives from the Anglo-Saxon word meaning "to lull". Alternatively, try *fennel* or *peppermint*.

point of view, the period of separation from his or her mother and father, which can sometimes cause anxiety at bedtime, is reduced when they all share a bed and he or she can fall asleep feeling more secure, knowing that they will not be alone for long. Children who co-sleep with parents also suffer fewer night-time disturbances such as sleepwalking or nightmares. By sharing a bed with their child (or children), parents gain peace of mind, and so sleep better, while reinforcing the emotional bond between the generations through physical proximity.

SLEEP AND THE NEW BABY

✻

The first few months after the birth of a new baby are a wonderful but exhausting time, when your sleep pattern inevitably becomes disrupted. If you are feeling fatigued, do not try to keep yourself awake by drinking beverages containing caffeine, such as tea and coffee, as once the stimulant's effects wear off you will feel even more tired (and if you are breast-feeding, some of the caffeine will enter your milk and keep the baby awake too). Also avoid alcohol and any drugs (including sedatives) if you are nursing your baby or co-sleeping. Instead, try some of the tips below on how to maximize sleep during this challenging period.

• Sleep whenever you can — instead of trying to catch up with housework, correspondence and so on, join your baby for a sleep during the day • If you are a working mother, nap with your baby at weekends • Try to go to bed immediately after nursing your baby — you will have a better chance of getting some deep sleep before the baby wakes for his or her next feed • Although you may feel tired during the day, try to stay busy — undertake gentle but engaging activities and try not to fall asleep unexpectedly.

Breastfeeding mothers in particular benefit from co-sleeping with their babies as they do not need to get up several times in the night to comfort a hungry and distressed child. They can just latch the infant on to feed at the first murmur and drift back to sleep. And even the father's sleep is less disturbed because the mother soon learns to provide the baby's feed before the infant starts to cry.

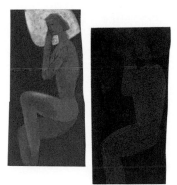

One of the main fears of parents who would like to share a bed with their baby is that they will inadvertently roll onto the child and cause injury. Research has shown that such worries are groundless, as parents seem to be instinctively aware of the infant's presence and automatically restrict their movements accordingly. However, anyone under the influence of alcohol or drugs, including some prescribed medications, should never co-sleep with their child. Consult your doctor if you are unsure.

Bear in mind that you will probably need less bedding when your child is with you in bed, as there will be increased warmth from his or her body heat. Be careful not to let newborn infants become too hot, as they are unable to regulate their own temperature by kicking off the covers.

Co-sleeping with a child does not require any equipment, but it might be wise to invest in an extra-wide mattress. It is easier and safer to lay the mattress on the ground, so that the baby cannot roll off the bed. This arrangement also allows you to expand the sleeping area by adding a mattress alongside the main one when the infant grows larger, or if you have another child. When the child decides that he or she wishes to sleep on their own (usually from two years old onward), you can gradually move the extra mattress further away.

Light and the Spectrum

The two properties of light – intensity and colour – influence sleep in different ways. Light intensity does not affect the sleeper directly, but its main impact is determined by our habits and how we originally learned to sleep. For example, if we are used to going to sleep in the dark, we will sleep better with the lights off, and vice versa. These indirect effects of light on sleep are modulated by the biological clock (see pp.30–31), the hormone melatonin (see pp.28–9), and their influence on the body's cycles.

Drapes or shades (blinds) are probably the most important bedroom furnishings as far as our sleep is concerned. By keeping out the sunlight in the early hours (especially in summer months), window coverings permit us to trick our biological clocks so that we can regulate our sleep patterns in line with the needs of our daily routines. Choose dark-coloured drapes or shades and ensure that they are fully lined to keep out all traces of light. Try to ensure that drapes have enough width in them to meet in the middle without leaving gaps at either end, and select shades that fully close together, blocking out all light.

Colours can have a strong effect on mood, so it is important that those we feature in our own bedrooms encourage rest. We vary in the way we respond to colour, but generally most of us find reds and yellows exciting and blues and greens relaxing. Because our response is individual, you need to discover your own most restful hues (see opposite). You could also paint the bedroom in neutral tones, such as white, which will not influence the impact of added colour, and then vary the tones of linen, rugs and cushions until you find the most relaxing hues.

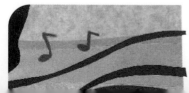

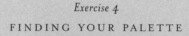

Exercise 4

FINDING YOUR PALETTE

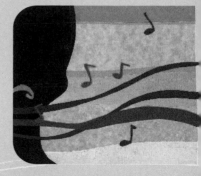

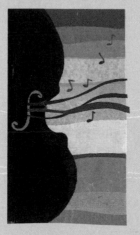

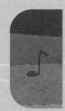

Colours vibrate (like sounds) at particular frequencies that affect our wellbeing. So, it is not surprising that certain types of music evoke certain colours in the mind of the listener. This exercise helps you pinpoint which colours make you feel most sleepy. (You will need some white paper and coloured pencils or crayons.)

1. Pick out pieces of music from your collection that promote each of the following moods: happy, inspired, excited, meditative, melancholic, reflective.

2. Each evening, listen to one piece of the music you selected. As your mood responds to the sounds, express your feelings with the pencils or crayons. (If you are not artistic, you can just draw blocks of the colours.) For example, perhaps the "Hallelujah Chorus" from Handel's Messiah *makes you draw red, or* Bridge Over Troubled Water *by Simon and Garfunkel brings the colour blue to mind. Continue to express yourself in this way until the music finishes.*

3. After you finish drawing, note on the back of the paper the mood you were in before you played the music, the feeling you thought the music would evoke, and how listening to it actually made you feel.

4. When you have listened to all your musical mood-categories, review your drawings. Which colours make you feel most relaxed?

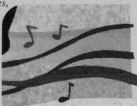

Feng Shui in the Bedroom

The ancient Chinese art of Feng Shui (pronounced "fung shway") draws upon the philosophical belief that our health, wellbeing and prosperity can be enhanced by harmonizing the invisible but powerful universal energy (*qi*) that flows throughout our environment. Literally meaning "wind-water" (the elements that the Chinese believed first carved out the land), Feng Shui has been practised in the East for several millennia and has now become highly popular in the West.

Originally, Feng Shui was used to find the most auspicious burial sites for the dead (this specialist Feng Shui practice is termed Yin Zhai). However, the modern practice of Feng Shui draws upon the general ancient principle that by balancing two complementary yet opposing elemental forces, known as *yin* and *yang*, we can harmonize *qi* in our environment (a practice specifically termed Yang Zhai). While *yin* is regarded as the passive, dark, feminine force, *yang* is the dynamic, light, masculine energy. It is particularly important to balance *yin* and *yang* in the bedroom as our sleep surroundings need to be both relaxing (*yin*) to encourage sleep and energizing (*yang*) to invigorate us upon waking.

According to the principles of Feng Shui, your bedroom should be a regular shape (ideally a square or a rectangle), simply decorated and free from clutter. Try sitting on your bed and examining the room. Can you see any items that have no business in a sleeping environment – a computer, for example, or outdoor coats hanging on the back of the door? Remove anything that you think does not belong there. Clothes and toiletries

Exercise 5
CLAPPING OUT TRAPPED *QI*

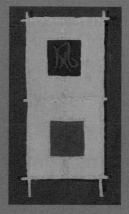

Trapped *qi* in the bedroom creates an imbalance of *yin* and *yang*, which adversely affects our sleep. *Qi* might become trapped under the bed and bed covers, in wardrobes and drawers and in the corners of the room. One space-clearing technique used by Feng Shui practitioners is "clapping out" such stagnant energy.

1. Look around your bedroom. Try to assess any areas where qi *might become trapped — look especially for corners formed not just by two abutting walls but by items of furniture against walls. Similarly, look for gaps under furniture.*

2. Begin at the entrance and work your way round the room anticlockwise. When you come to a corner formed by walls, face it and raise your hands above your head. Clap gently (the bedroom, a peaceful space, needs soft claps) twice, then lower your arms to chest height and clap gently twice again. Repeat at waist level and then move on to the next qi *trap. Clap down the height of corners formed by furniture and walls; and crouch down and clap gently at the mouths of gaps under items of furniture. Open wardrobes or drawers and clap inside.*

3. At the bed, pull back the covers and clap twice at the head, middle and foot of each side of the bed. Crouch down and clap gently under the bed on each side.

4. Once you have finished, wash your hands under running cold water — this will remove the static build-up of stagnant energy on your hands.

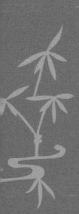

should be stored in cupboards and kept out of sight as much as possible to reduce visual over-stimulation. You should avoid having mirrors on the walls (try putting them on the inside of your wardrobe doors instead), unless your bedroom is not square or rectangular, in which case a mirror should be placed to reflect an angle into the space where a corner is missing. If you need a mirror in your bedroom, try not to place it opposite the bed as it will reflect energy back at you while you sleep. The bed itself should be raised off the floor on legs, rather than being flat on the floor like a futon mattress, to encourage a balanced flow of *qi* around the sleeping area. Try to position the bed so that as you lie in it you are able to see people entering the room.

Feng Shui also has guidelines on placing your bed in certain energy fields. Vital energy is said to flow directly between windows and doors, and also in the area between two doors — try not to place your bed in either of these spaces as the energy there will disrupt your sleep. Although we may enjoy the luxury of an *en suite* bathroom, in Feng Shui this is considered disruptive. If you do have an *en suite*, avoid positioning your bed between the door to the *en suite* and the bedroom door — otherwise your bed will be in the path of another field of conflicting energy, one cleansing, one restful. Ideally, use a moveable screen to block the energy between the two entrances — although this may impracticably reduce the space available in the room. If direct sunlight falls across the bed during the day, try to move the bed to a more shaded position — the energy of the sun is inappropriate for a sleeping surface.

It is inadvisable to have anything, such as a picture or bookshelf, hanging on the wall above the head of your bed. To encourage good sleep, the area around where your head will lie should be kept completely uncluttered. If you live in a studio apartment, where sleeping and living space are combined, make the area immediately surrounding the bed a special space, free from objects that serve the other uses of the room.

The final factor thought to have considerable impact on both the quality and duration of our sleep is the direction in which your head points as you lie in bed. On the following pages you will find a Pa Kua chart, which will help you to work out the best way for your head to point, and to adjust the position of your bed accordingly.

THE POWER OF EARTH ENERGY

When we try to improve our sleep by changing the position of our bed it is important to take into account the energy that emanates from the land below our building. Some Feng Shui practitioners believe that this energy, known as *geopathic stress*, can have a considerable effect on both our sleep and our wellbeing. If our bed is positioned over places where the earth's energy lines cross (and as a consequence electromagnetic fields build up), we might suffer from sleep disturbances, such as sleepwalking or nightmares. But people who are especially sensitive to geopathic stress often experience minor sleep disruptions. For example, they may find that they habitually wake up in one particular corner of the bed, as they instinctively move away from an energy field. Often such problems can be solved simply by moving the bed, but if sleep is severely disrupted, it may be advisable to call in a professional dowser to pinpoint the problematic areas.

The Pa Kua Chart

For optimal sleep, Feng Shui experts stress the importance of sleeping with your head in the correct position – if you sleep oriented toward the most auspicious direction according to the Chinese laws of the zodiac, you will maximize your potential for good health and wellbeing. To discover your best direction (known as *sheng chi*) use the Pa Kua chart opposite, which is based on the Pa Kua octagon of eight compass points, each of which governs a specific area of life – for example, the north point governs successful relationships.

First identify your year of birth in the Chinese Horoscope table. (Most birth years correspond with the Western calendar, but if your birthday falls between January 1 and February 20, you need to check the date of the Chinese New Year in the year of your birth – you can find this information on specialist Chinese astrology websites.) The animal name at the top of the column in which your year of birth is located gives you your Chinese sign of the zodiac. For example, a girl born in May 1975 will be a rabbit as she was born in the Year of the Rabbit. Still focusing on the girl's year of birth, look across to the far left-hand column and note the number that appears there – it is 6. Turning to the Kua table, we now look up number 6, for women, under the rabbit column, which gives us her Kua number – 8. Finally, to find the girl's *sheng chi* direction, we consult the *sheng chi* table. We look under the number 8 and this shows that for both sexes the best direction in which to sleep is with the head pointing to the southwest.

CHINESE HOROSCOPE *Finding your Chinese sign of the zodiac*

	Rat	Ox	Tiger	Rabbit	Dragon	Snake	Horse	Sheep	Monkey	Rooster	Dog	Boar
1	1912	1913	1914	1915	1916	1917	1918	1919	1920	1921	1922	1923
2	1924	1925	1926	1927	1928	1929	1930	1931	1932	1933	1934	1935
3	1936	1937	1938	1939	1940	1941	1942	1943	1944	1945	1946	1947
4	1948	1949	1950	1951	1952	1953	1954	1955	1956	1957	1958	1959
5	1960	1961	1962	1963	1964	1965	1966	1967	1968	1969	1970	1971
6	1972	1973	1974	1975	1976	1977	1978	1979	1980	1981	1982	1983
7	1984	1985	1986	1987	1988	1989	1990	1991	1992	1993	1994	1995
8	1996	1997	1998	1999	2000	2001	2002	2003	2004	2005	2006	2007

KUA NUMBERS *Determining your spiritual number*

		Rat	Ox	Tiger	Rabbit	Dragon	Snake	Horse	Sheep	Monkey	Rooster	Dog	Boar
Men	1	7	6	5	4	3	2	1	9	8	7	6	5
Women	1	8	9	1	2	3	4	5	6	7	8	9	1
Men	2	4	3	2	1	9	8	7	6	5	4	3	2
Women	2	2	3	4	5	6	7	8	9	1	2	3	4
Men	3	1	9	8	7	6	5	4	3	2	1	9	8
Women	3	5	6	7	8	9	1	2	3	4	5	6	7
Men	4	7	6	5	4	3	2	1	9	8	7	6	5
Women	4	8	9	1	2	3	4	5	6	7	8	9	1
Men	5	4	3	2	1	9	8	7	6	5	4	3	2
Women	5	2	3	4	5	6	7	8	9	1	2	3	4
Men	6	1	9	8	7	6	5	4	3	2	1	9	8
Women	6	5	6	7	8	9	1	2	3	4	5	6	7
Men	7	7	6	5	4	3	2	1	9	8	7	6	5
Women	7	8	9	1	2	3	4	5	6	7	8	9	1
Men	8	4	3	2	1	9	8	7	6	5	4	3	2
Women	8	2	3	4	5	6	7	8	9	1	2	3	4

SHENG CHI *The best direction for sleep*

Kua Number	1	2	3	4	5	6	7	8	9
ALL	SE	NE	S	N		W	NW	SW	E
MEN					NE				
WOMEN					SW				

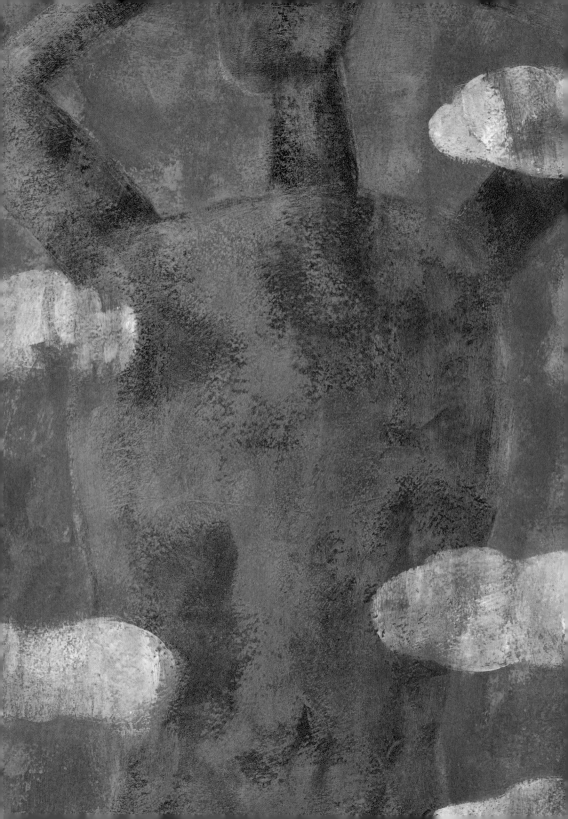

The Sleeping Body

We have seen that one of the possible reasons why we sleep is to allow our body time to repair and refresh itself so that we function well the following day. However, modern lifestyles in the West have disturbed our natural sleep patterns. Instead of following nature's cycle of sleeping when it is dark and waking when it becomes light, we use artificial lighting to stay active well into the hours of darkness. Our workplace is often a stressful environment and, as many of us find no time to relax, we go to bed exhausted and tense. If we take into account other factors that are detrimental to our health, such as poor diet, smoking, and a high consumption of caffeine and alcohol, we have a recipe for almost certain insomnia.

In this chapter we explore how to make our behaviour more sleep-friendly. By examining topics such as diet, exercise and physical relaxation techniques, both Eastern and Western, we learn how to adopt a healthier, more harmonious lifestyle, which will enable us to obtain plenty of the deep, restorative sleep we need to live life to the full.

Sustenance for Sleep

Eating increases our metabolic rate and causes our body temperature to rise — in other words, it energizes us. We already know that the perfect time for us to try to go to sleep is as our body temperature is dropping — a process which usually begins about an hour before our normal bedtime. It stands to reason, then, that if we eat shortly before we intend to go to bed, our ability to fall asleep may be badly affected. However, we might also know from practical experience that a large meal at lunchtime makes us feel sleepy in the afternoon (this is because eating when our body temperature is high causes the brain to divert energy away from the muscles to work the digestive system, which makes us feel sluggish). So, if we are to get the right amount of sleep at the right time, when should we eat? The rules are straightforward: try to avoid having one big meal at the end of the day — and certainly try not to eat a main meal later than

SWEET DREAMS

Why not try the following delicious nightcap made with milk, which contains the natural sleep-promoting chemical tryptophan. Place 8 fluid ounces (200 ml) of milk in a small saucepan. Stir in one teaspoon of ground cinnamon and bring the mixture to the boil. Simmer for a couple of minutes. Pour into a mug, add honey to sweeten, if necessary, and drink immediately.

three hours before you intend to go to bed. Aim to eat little and often, rather than having one light and one heavy meal a day (or two heavy meals) — this will keep your metabolism on a fairly even keel and the food's effects on your ability to sleep (or to stay awake!) should be minimalized.

Once we have looked at our eating routines, we should assess how the food we eat might affect how we sleep. Certain foods do have a particular reputation for either disturbing or promoting sleep. Take cheese — the popular belief is that it caus- 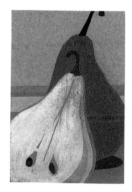 es nightmares. Scientific evidence shows that there is indeed a link, because tyramine, an ingredient in cheese, increases the level of chemicals that cause high blood pressure, which is a stress symptom asso- ciated with nightmares. Conversely, lettuce was used by the ancient Egyptians for its soporific and pain- killing properties. But, despite the fact that recent research confirms the presence of a painkilling opi- ate in lettuce leaves, the amounts are so low that its effects on sleep are likely to be minimal.

The food that we eat has far-reaching implications in all aspects of our lives. If we eat unhealthily, we can suffer from heartburn, indigestion and numerous other food-related disor- ders, which can affect our sleep adversely. Eating to improve sleep is about ensuring that we eat healthily in general, not just to enhance the part of our lives that we spend sleeping.

Try to make sure that you obtain a full complement of vita- mins from your food. In particular some researchers believe that a lack of vitamin B-complex (especially niacin, pantothenic acid, B_6 and B_{12}) in the diet can lead to sleep problems. If you are a meat-eater, try to eat lean cuts of pork, lamb and veal. If you prefer to eat fish, trout and sardines contain a variety of

B-complex vitamins too. Chicken, tuna, and fortified breakfast cereals are good sources of niacin; broad beans are rich in pantothenic acid; wheatgerm, turbot, walnuts and baked potatoes contain Vitamin B_6, and Vitamin B_{12} is found in yogurt, cheese and seaweed.

Research has shown that the mineral magnesium can significantly affect the quality of our sleep. One study proved that eating foods containing high amounts of magnesium resulted in an improved night's sleep with fewer awakenings. Green vegetables, avocados, bananas, peanut butter, nuts and seeds are all good sources of this vital mineral.

Eat organic! Many foods we eat contain harmful additives that can injuriously affect our sleep. *Monosodium glutamate* (MSG), for example, often found in processed foods and fast Oriental foods, is known to cause digestive upsets, heartburn, headaches and many other disorders that can affect our sleep. (Note that apart from being an additive, MSG is also found naturally in mushrooms, carrots and some seaweeds.) Another additive to avoid is the yellow colouring *tartrazine* (E-102), found widely in fizzy drinks, cookies and candy — it has been linked with hyperactivity in children and is thought to trigger asthma, eczema, rashes and other irritations in susceptible people.

Of course, it is not only what we eat that affects our overall wellbeing, and therefore, our sleep, but what we drink, too. Apart from avoiding the substances that are obviously detrimental to sleep, such as caffeine (see pp.78–9), we should remember that our body requires three to four pints (1.7 to 2.3 litres) of water a day to replace fluids that are naturally lost every 24 hours. Unfortunately, most of us rarely drink anywhere near that much

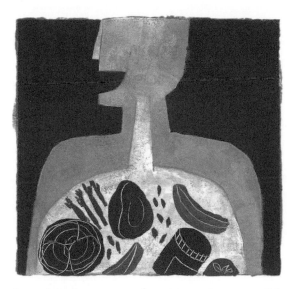

water, and yet dehydration is often ignored as a possible cause of a bad night's sleep. Think how often you wake up in the morning feeling lethargic and thirsty. Many of us even wake during the night to go to the kitchen for a glass of water.

Over the next three days, why not conduct a little experiment? Make a conscious effort to drink between three and four pints (1.7 to 2.3 litres) of water each day, at regular intervals, commencing tomorrow (but make sure that you start early in the day because otherwise you may find yourself waking up to go the bathroom during the night!). As you do the experiment, note down in your sleep journal how you felt on waking each morning. Do you feel brighter and less lethargic? Is your head "clearer"? Even if something else is affecting your sleep and drinking more water seems to have little or no effect, you will be replenishing your body with the essential fluids it needs to function at an optimal level, and this will improve your overall health and wellbeing, which in turn will have a beneficial effect on your sleep.

Catching Sleep Thieves

Drinking beverages such as coffee, tea and cola, having a couple of beers or glasses of wine and a smoke to help us wind down, are accepted social behaviours in modern life in the West. But how many of us realize that between them these drinks, and cigarettes, contain the three main "sleep thieves" — caffeine, alcohol and nicotine — which are powerful compounds that stimulate or depress the brain and have a considerable impact on our sleep.

Many people would feel lost without a cup of coffee or tea to kick-start their day. The stimulating action of these beverages is caused by the chemical **caffeine** (tea contains less caffeine than coffee, but enough to make us feel "awake") which activates the wakefulness centres in the brain, making us more mentally alert and also increasing our physical powers of endurance. But the more caffeine we consume, the more tolerant to it we become, and the more caffeine we need to obtain the same level of alertness. Conversely, if we ration our intake, the little that we do consume becomes more effective.

Caffeine remains in the body for several hours — and up to five times longer in pregnant women. If we have a lot of coffee over the course of a day, caffeine can have a cumulative effect that makes it difficult for us to both fall and remain sleep. To ensure that caffeine does not disturb your sleep, it is best to avoid drinks containing this chemical for ten hours before bedtime. If you really cannot do without your morning boost, limit your intake to one or two beverages early in the day.

However, if you really wish to improve your sleep, it is wise to consider adopting a caffeine-free regime from the middle of the day onward. If you fear that you will really miss the taste of coffee and tea, do not despair — decaffeinated brands are now widely available. Or you could try herbal drinks, such as dandelion-root coffee, or teas, such as rosehip, peppermint and fennel (see also below), which are healthier, chemical-free alternatives. If you normally drink lots of cola and other carbonated drinks, substitute fizzy mineral water instead; in so doing, you will beneficially increase your water consumption.

While hot and cold drinks containing caffeine act as stimulants, **alcohol** has the opposite effect. Most of us drink occasionally at social events, or we may have a small tipple every evening to help us relax. While a small amount, such as a glass of wine, can have a calming effect, a larger quantity of alcohol can interfere with the quality of our sleep by reducing the amount of deep and REM sleep that we obtain. After consuming alcohol, it is not uncommon to wake up periodically perspiring heavily, experiencing palpitations and generally feeling restless.

A HERBAL TEA FOR SLEEP

Although you can buy herb teas from supermarkets and health-food stores, why not make your own infusion to help you sleep? Choose one to three of the following, mixing any combination: hops, valerian, camomile, passion flowers, skullcap, lemon balm. Steep the herbs in hot water for five minutes. Drink this tea in the early evening to give it time to work before you go to bed.

Let us assume that you have decided to give up alcohol altogether to improve your sleep. You will need to devise a strategy to help you resist temptation at parties, receptions and visits to bars with friends or work colleagues. Choose alcohol-free wines, beers or fruit juices, or drink mineral water, but take care to avoid caffeine-rich colas and sodas containing additives that can affect sleep. Some bars and restaurants also offer a range of non-alcoholic cocktails, freshly made to order, that contain health-promoting natural fruit juices.

If you usually have an alcoholic "nightcap" before going to bed to help you sleep, examine your underlying motive. Think back to when you first started doing this. What was happening in your life at the time? Was it because you were depressed or having emotional problems? Perhaps your circumstances have now changed and you are only drinking before bedtime because it has become a habit. If this is the case, substitute a hot milky drink or herbal tea, which promotes sleep. But if problems with sleeplessness persist, perhaps you could try a different approach. Instead of using alcohol as a prop, you might arrange to telephone a sympathetic friend or close family member to discuss your worries before you go to bed. Airing your difficulties in this way should help to restore your peace of mind and so aid sleep.

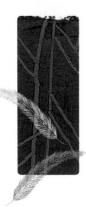

The third of our sleep thieves is **nicotine**, the stimulant we inhale with every puff of tobacco smoke. Although the initial effect of the nicotine is to make smokers feel more alert, this does not last long and they invariably feel relaxed shortly after having a cigarette. This may give them the erroneous impression that smoking can help them sleep. Unfortunately, what smokers are experiencing as relaxation is really the satisfaction gained from quenching an addictive

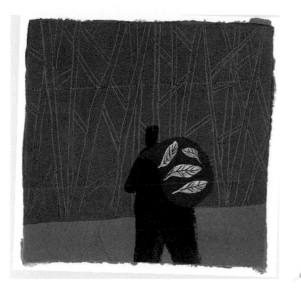

craving for nicotine. They may fall asleep but, as soon as the nicotine is metabolized, the brain wakes up the smoker to remind them that they need more. Nicotine also triggers the release of epinephrine (adrenaline), the body's stress response, stopping us from getting our required quota of deep sleep.

Proof that our sleep suffers from smoking is shown in recent research from Pennsylvania State University, which found that smokers took approximately twice as long to fall asleep as non-smokers. However, interestingly, within two nights of giving up, the time it took the ex-smokers to go to sleep fell from an average of 52 to eighteen minutes.

There is no such thing as a "best" way to kick the habit — there are many different methods. For example, you could gradually cut down on cigarettes, substitute them with nicotine patches or gum, or you could try an alternative approach such as hypnotherapy or acupuncture. Help yourself by avoiding situations in which you usually smoke, and ban smoking in bed or in the bedroom, especially just before you go to sleep.

Fitness for Sleep

Our bodies are designed for vigorous action, but if we lead a sedentary life, sitting at a desk for most of the day or spending hours in a car, the natural range of our movements becomes restricted, with consequences for our wellbeing. If we spend long periods in one position, tension builds up in our muscles. Then, when we try to sleep at night, this accumulated physical stress makes us restless and uneasy — our body cannot relax. This is the beginning of a cycle of sleeplessness: we cannot sleep so we lie awake worrying about the fact that we cannot sleep (and compounding the problem by adding psychological stress), so we become even more tense, and so it goes on. It would not be an exaggeration, then, to say that some insomnia is caused simply because we do not move our bodies often or energetically enough during the day. However, there is a simple remedy to release tension and help you sleep — it is called exercise!

But if the mere thought of exercise makes you shudder, it is worth remembering that it has gentle forms which do not require you to push your body to its physical limits. For example, someone suffering from a build-up of tension can benefit greatly from gentle stretching (see opposite) before going to bed. Or, you can incorporate exercise into your daily routine at work and stop the build-up of stresses before they accumulate. If you habitually take the elevator in your office building, start using the stairs instead. You can begin by walking down, just one flight, then increase it to two, and so on. Once you feel good about walking down to the bottom, you can set yourself the more demanding challenge of walking up. The

Exercise 6

THE PRE-SLEEP STRETCH

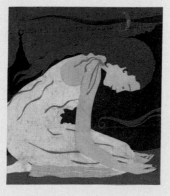

Exercise need not be vigorous to be beneficial. A sedentary lifestyle can adversely affect our posture and we often find ourselves complaining of aching necks and stiff backs. As much of the tension of daily life is stored in your spine, a pre-sleep exercise that stretches this area can help to relieve any tightness there, and so help you to fall asleep more easily and to avoid waking up during the night, or in the morning, with muscular pain.

1. Kneel, with the tops of your feet flat on the floor, and sit back on your heels. Bend forward, stretching your arms out in front of you and "folding" your upper body over your thighs until your forehead touches the floor. Swing your arms round so that they lie beside your body, the palms of your hands facing upwards. Breathe deeply and slowly for one minute.

2. Move up onto all fours, with your hands at shoulders' width apart and your knees directly beneath your hips. Inhale, lift your head up and at the same time push your bottom outward, dipping your back in a cat-like stretch. Exhale and breathe rhythmically, holding the position for approximately 30 seconds.

3. Inhale, and lower your head as if to look between your legs. As you exhale, tuck your chin into your chest. Arch your back upward and tuck in your bottom. Breathing rhythmically, stay in this position for approximately 30 seconds.

4. Move back into the Step-1 position; breathe deeply and slowly for one minute.

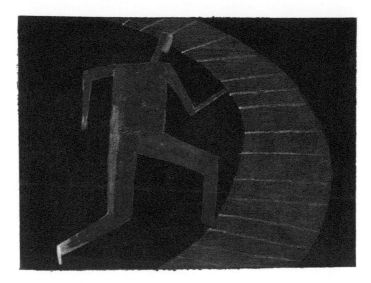

important thing is to make a start. However, if you are over-weight, have heart problems, or suffer from any other medical condition, you should consult your doctor before embarking on any exercise regime. Remember to "listen" to your body and respond sensibly to its needs.

Physical exercise interacts with sleep by affecting the body's metabolic rate and temperature in much the same way as diet (see pp.74–7). The various metabolic and hormonal changes associated with vigorous exercise are stimulating and boost the body's temperature. Sleep comes more easily when our temperature is decreasing and, if we wish to use exercise to enhance our sleep, it makes sense to finish any strenuous workouts by late afternoon. Early research showed that walking on a treadmill during the day promoted sleep that night, but only if undertaken at least five or six hours before going to bed. The state of relaxation we experience after exercising also helps us to obtain our full quota of deep sleep (see pp.40–41).

So how much exercise do we need to do to improve our sleep? It is probably less than you think — three sessions of twenty minutes each per week will do the trick, provided that you do aerobic exercise, which boosts your oxygen consumption, improves your breathing and strengthens your heart and circulation — all benefits to your health that will help you sleep better.

The most important thing to remember is that any exercise regime will help to improve your sleep, as long as during exercise you hit your heart rate "target zone". To find out what this is, subtract your age from 220 to get the advised maximum exercising heart rate for someone of your age. Then calculate 60 and 75 per cent of this figure, which gives the lower and upper limits of the target range for your heart rate during exercise. For example, if you are aged 35, 220-35=185 — your maximum heart rate per minute; 60 and 75 per cent of this figure are 111 and 138 respectively, so your target heart rate during exercise is between 111 and 138 beats per minute. Any aerobic exercise, such as cycling, swimming, jogging and so on, that raises your heart rate within the target zone for twenty minutes, is suitable. You can monitor your heart rate during exercise by resting, taking your pulse for one minute and counting the number of heartbeats.

Choose an activity or sport that you enjoy, as this will provide an incentive to keep up the exercise program. And be flexible — if you get bored with swimming and so on, there are suggestions for other gentle forms of exercise you might like to try on the following pages. But whatever activity you undertake, do not overdo things and always add on an extra five-minute warm-up period before starting and another five minutes afterwards to cool down — otherwise you risk injuring yourself, and pain is certainly no aid to better sleep!

The Indian Path

Yoga is an ancient Indian tradition that balances the body's vital energy, or *prana*, through a mixture of postures, breathing exercises and meditation. This long-established practice has become popular in the West as a discipline that promotes good health and personal development. Yoga is open to anyone, of any age and level of fitness, and its non-competitive nature allows participants to progress at their own pace. While it is always better to learn from a qualified teacher, it is possible to do some of the basic exercises on your own.

Sleep problems are almost unknown among *yogis* – advanced practitioners of yoga. So what is their secret? Unfortunately, there is no magic formula, but the key to improving our quality of sleep through yoga lies in adopting postures, or *asanas*, and doing breathing exercises, known as *pranayama*, which together help us to relax and release mental, as well as physical, tension.

A typical session of Hatha Yoga – the type most widely practised in the West – consists of a warm-up, followed by several postures to stretch every part of the body, and then a period of relaxation in which breath control plays an essential part. One of the simplest and most useful postures is the *Shavasana* or Corpse Pose, which is often used at the beginning and end of yoga sessions. Lie flat on your back, arms at your sides, palms facing upwards with your feet about two feet (50cm) apart. Close your eyes and breathe deeply. Roll your head from side to side so that first one ear and then the other touches the ground. Then bring your head back to the centre and focus on your breathing for at least five minutes or until you feel completely relaxed.

Exercise 7

BREATHING AWAY STRESS

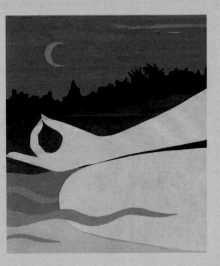

After a stressful day, use this exercise, which combines breathing and arm movements, to banish tension and relax your body ready for sleep. Performed 20 minutes before bedtime, it will help you to establish slow and regular breathing for a good night's sleep.

1. Sit in a chair with your arms loose by your sides, eyes closed. Switch off the part of your mind that analyzes your thoughts and try to banish mental clutter. Focus on the rhythm of your breath for two to three minutes.

2. Inhaling gently, raise your arms slightly, cross them in front of your body and bring them up over your head, uncrossing them as you go. Now exhale and swoop your arms down to your sides again. The whole movement should be executed in one long, circular sweep. Repeat four times.

3. Inhale and raise your arms outwards and upwards touching your fingertips above your head. Exhale as you lower your arms. Repeat three times.

4. Inhale, stretching your arms out parallel in front of you. Keep them straight, and raise them above your head. Exhale, lowering your arms. Repeat twice.

The Chinese Traditions

In Chinese medicine, sleeplessness is thought to arise through an imbalance in the flow of *qi* (energy), which is channelled to the major organs of the body along twelve pathways called meridians. The flow of *qi* is created by the interplay between two forces, *yin* and *yang*, which can be thought of as opposite yet complementary aspects of the universal principle – for example, dark and light, female and male, and so on. However, nothing is entirely *yin* nor wholly *yang* – a seed of one principle is always contained within the other.

The twelve major organs of the body (corresponding to the twelve meridians) are divided into six *yin* and six *yang*. While normal sleep is composed of alternating cycles of *yin* and *yang*, disturbed sleep is caused by an imbalance of these two principles in a particular organ. For example, restlessness at night, causing us continually to wake and fall asleep again, suggests a Kidney imbalance; frequent early waking indicates a Gall Bladder disharmony; and sleep disrupted by vivid dreams suggests either a Liver or Heart imbalance. The Chinese have developed a wide range of exercises, which can be used to balance *yin* and *yang* in our bodies and to regulate the flow of *qi*. In the following pages we explore some of the traditions that can aid our sleep, such as the ancient arts of T'ai Chi, Qigong and acupressure.

The Chinese discipline of T'ai Chi is a form of moving meditation, which both improves the circulation of the body's vital energy and focuses the mind. Its combination of physical and mental exercise can be particularly useful in helping us to sleep, as it relieves physical tension by relaxing our muscles and also calms the mind. The movements and rhythm in T'ai Chi exercises also promote balance, alignment of the body, precise muscle control and suppleness.

It is thought that an early form of T'ai Chi was invented in the sixth century by Bodhidharma, an Indian monk, who created a combination of meditation and movement to improve the poor physical health of his fellow monks. The first thirteen T'ai Chi postures and attitudes were devised at the turn of the fourteenth century as static positions, which subsequently evolved into a series of continuous movements. Although T'ai Chi developed into a martial art during the seventeenth century, its focus has remained on the mind and relaxation, rather than on force and strength. It requires no special equipment and the movements can be performed by anyone, regardless of age or physical aptitude. Today, in China, large groups of people practise T'ai Chi outdoors, first thing in the morning, to help them prepare for the day. But there are also T'ai Chi movements that are more suitably performed in the evening to aid relaxation.

One quick and simple exercise that you might try concentrates on relaxing the shoulders and arms and, for optimum results, should be practised approximately one hour before going to bed. Standing with your feet at shoulders' width apart, rest your left hand on your left shoulder and your right hand on your right shoulder. Now make circling movements with your elbows, starting with thirty seconds of forward rotations, followed by another thirty seconds of backward ones. Then, raise your arms parallel to the floor. Stretch your hands out in front of you and slowly raise your right arm as high as you can, while at the same time lowering your left arm to your side. Hold this position for ten seconds, before repeating with the arms in the opposite positions. Do this whole sequence of movements twice.

Another Chinese discipline that is growing in popularity in the West is Qigong, which many people approach initially through an interest in T'ai Chi. In fact, T'ai Chi is regarded by some as being essentially a moving form of Qigong, as the two disciplines have much the same basic principles. The practice of Qigong began in China more than 5,000 years ago. Since then it has been developed and refined by Buddhist and Daoist scholars, and doctors and practitioners of the martial arts.

Qigong can help to promote better sleep by harmonizing the body's qi, using a combination of physical movement and postures, breath control, and meditation techniques. Why not try a relaxation exercise that strengthens the flow of qi in the kidneys — an area where imbalances particularly affect our sleep (the kidneys are located on either side of the spine, above the waist and behind the lower ribs). Try lying on your back on the floor, bending your right leg upward and outward, resting your foot against the inside of your left knee. Place your left hand, palm up, under your left kidney, and your right hand, palm down, over your navel. Now imagine that your left hand is warming your kidney and that energy from your right hand enters your body through the navel to your left kidney. Do the same again (left leg bent), warming your right kidney with your right hand.

The ancient art of acupressure can also be useful in the treatment of insomnia. Based on the same principles as acupuncture, acupressure is a technique in which vital energy points, known as acupoints, are pressed or massaged with the thumbs, or the middle or index fingers, to balance the body's qi. Acupressure can be used by anyone as a self-help measure, or as a form of Chinese "first aid" if carried out by a partner or friend. Try the exercise opposite, in which the acupoints most effective in the promotion of good sleep are massaged.

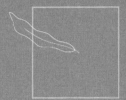

Exercise 8

ACUPRESSURE FOR SLEEP

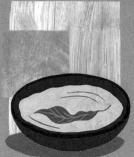

Try the following acupressure exercise one hour before going to bed each night, then again immediately before you try to go to sleep. Do this for at least two weeks – longer if possible – to give yourself a chance to notice the full improvement to your sleep.

1. Starting with your head, and using the fingertips of your middle and index fingers, press the top of the centre of your skull for approximately 30 seconds.

2. Using your index fingertips, make small circular movements simultaneously at the outer ends of your eyebrows for 30 seconds. Next, using the pads of your thumbs, wipe the upper, followed by the lower, edges of your eyesockets, from the inner to the outer corners. Then, rub the palms of your hands together until they feel warm, and place them over your eyes for 45 seconds. Finish working on the eye area by lightly resting the heels of your hands on your closed eyelids for 30 seconds.

3. Supporting your left hand in your right hand (both hands palm up), find the acupressure point (known as Heart 7) located on the crease of your wrist in line with your little finger. Press and release this spot with the tip of your thumb for roughly a minute. Repeat the same procedure on your right wrist.

4. Find the acupoint located between the tendons, approximately 2 inches (5cm) above the left wrist on the inside of your left forearm, and make small, firm circular movements with your thumb for one minute. Repeat this kneading movement on the right wrist.

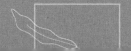

Baths for Sleep

According to the principles of Chinese hydrotherapy, sleep problems can be helped by taking a warm bath for fifteen to twenty minutes approximately half an hour before going to bed. It is thought that warm baths encourage both the smooth flow of *qi* and better blood circulation. Western sleep experiments endorse this claim, showing that warm baths taken just prior to bed indeed hasten sleep, particularly in the elderly. Adding herbs, such as camomile (which has sedative properties), to a bath can be especially effective. Infuse two teaspoonfuls of the herb in boiling water and leave the mixture to stand for ten minutes. Then pour it through a strainer into your bath water.

Chinese medicine warns against spending a long time in the bath or having the water temperature too high, as this can raise the body temperature, which is counter-productive to sleep. Although you may feel relaxed immediately after a hot bath, you may later feel thirsty and restless. Menopausal women, in particular, should avoid steamy baths, as the heat can trigger uncomfortable hot flushes and night sweats, which tend to disrupt sleep.

Another method of stabilizing the flow of *qi* and promoting sleep is the hydrotherapy footbath, which you can try just before bedtime. Fill two large bowls, one with hot (slightly hotter than your usual bathwater temperature), the other with cold water. Make sure that the water level reaches above your ankles. Place both your feet in the hot water for three minutes, and then immerse them in the cold water for thirty seconds. Repeat this procedure four times. Then, dry your feet and put on warm socks before going to bed.

Exercise 9

INHALING CALM

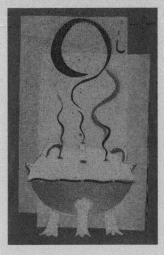

When you need to sleep particularly well — for example, on the eve of a job interview — try the following inhalation exercise, which is especially effective when you are relaxed after a bath. You will need some Eaglewood (*Lignum aquilariae agallochae*), which is renowned for its sleep-promoting effects when inhaled, and some incense charcoals — both can be purchased from Chinese herbal stores.

1. Prepare the Eaglewood by grinding it into a coarse powder, or by breaking it into small pieces. Place the charcoal in an incense burner or on an inflammable dish, and set it alight.

2. Sitting near the burner, sprinkle the Eaglewood onto the charcoal. Close your eyes and breathe deeply for two minutes as the fragrance of the aromatic wood is released around you.

3. Now open your eyes and lean over the charcoal (keeping your face approximately two feet/50cm above it) and gently inhale the smoke as it rises. Breathe deeply and rhythmically. After a few minutes you should feel a great sense of calm. Focus on this feeling of tranquillity for one minute.

4. Extinguish any remaining charcoal and go straight to bed.

Soothing Touch

When we wish to improve the quality of our sleep, we should consider a valuable, innate tool that we often overlook — the soothing power of touch. Since ancient times the laying-on of hands in massage has been used all over the world to promote healing, to help to restore balance in the body and to encourage refreshing, restorative sleep.

Human beings are tactile — even before we are born, we are sensitive to touch, and once we enter the world we continue to crave this most basic form of contact throughout our lives. But as the demands of busy life today do not always allow time for physical contact, we often become distanced from our loved ones, and both physical and emotional tension builds. Massage can provide an enjoyable, therapeutic way to relax each other.

Touching is instinctive. Even if we do not realize it, massage is something that we all know how to do. For example, if our child bumps him- or herself, our first reaction is to rub the affected area to ease the pain. And one of the simplest and most enjoyable ways to wind down with our partner, and to promote good sleep, is through mutual massage (see pp.58–9).

Think how often you put your hand on your opposite shoulder and knead or rub the area to relieve tightness — you, yourself, are the only person who knows the exact site of your tension. You may not realize it but this almost instinctive action is actually a form of self-massage. Although we usually perceive massage as something one person does to another, self-massage (see opposite) can be a useful tool to relieve tension in situations where another person is unavailable.

Exercise 10

STROKING AWAY TENSION

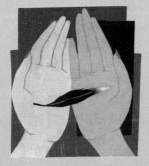

When you are stressed and tired from lack of sleep, the tell-tale signs show first in your face. Giving yourself a pre-sleep face massage can release tension and improve your appearance by increasing the circulation to the skin: not only will you sleep more deeply, you will also wake up feeling and looking refreshed.

1. Prepare by having a warm, soothing bath. Or put yourself in a tranquil mood by dimming the lights and listening to some relaxing music.

2. Sit on the floor or on a chair and support yourself with cushions so that you are comfortable.

3. With arms bent and out to the sides, put the index and middle fingers of both hands flat on your forehead between your hairline and eyebrows. Making small circular movements, rub your forehead for one to two minutes.

4. Using the same rotating movements, massage your temples, taking care to apply a lighter pressure to this sensitive area. Continue for one to two minutes.

5. Place your index and middle fingers on your cheekbones and rub them for one to two minutes, again using small circular movements. (This part of the massage is particularly helpful if you tend to clench your jaw or grind your teeth during sleep.)

6. Gently press your thumbs under the tops of your eyesockets on either side of your nose. Hold this position for approximately 10 seconds. Repeat five times.

Herbalism and Aromatherapy

Around 3000BCE, in Mesopotamia in the Near East, the world's first civilizations arose. Little is known of their healing practices but among the 30,000 surviving clay tablets there are approximately 1,000 which deal with herbal medicine; and herbs such as juniper, and oils such as cedar, are itemized.

The ancient Egyptians used the scents of specific plants during religious rituals to reach a higher level of consciousness or to promote tranquillity. More recently, in 1928, French chemist Henri Gattefosse introduced the word "aromathérapie". After an explosion badly burned his hand, Gattefosse plunged it into a vat of lavender, and noticed that the burns healed quickly, leaving little scarring. This spurred him into researching the therapeutic effects of lavender and other herbal oils.

Herbs tend not to be prescribed by herbalists as antidotes to illness, but more as triggers of various physiological functions that enable the body to heal itself. For sleep improvement this means using herbs to help the body to combat the ailments (mental or physical) that lead to sleeplessness; very often, of course, the cause might be anxiety, but aching limbs, colds or 'flu and upset stomachs also disrupt our sleep.

Taking herbal remedies can be enjoyable as well as practical — try making herbal infusions; place a few drops of the herbal essence in your bath; or use an oil burner and inhale the aroma as part of a pre-sleep relaxation exercise. Sufferers from insomnia in particular are thought to benefit by drinking herbal tea or using aromatherapy.

Many herbs are particularly associated with improving sleep or curing insomnia. Over this and the following two pages, we list some of the best-known and most effective of them, and how they are traditionally taken or used for sleep improvement. (Before taking or applying any of these remedies, it is best to consult a qualified herbalist or aromatherapist.)

CALIFORNIAN POPPY
This plant has a reputation for being a non-addictive alternative to the opium poppy. It was used by Native North Americans to relieve toothache. Known as a sedative, it is said to be useful for calming over-excitable children. It is used in infusions.

HOPS
Hop flowers are used extensively in the treatment of sleeplessness. An infusion is made for the relief of anxiety, stress and general pain. This plant reputedly acts as a tranquillizer, sedative and digestive aid and may also decrease our desire for alcohol. No formal comparisons have been made, but some herbalists

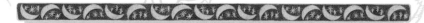

MAKING A HERBAL PILLOW
*

Some people find that a herbal pillow helps them to sleep. To make your own, fill a small fabric bag with lavender, orange peel and cloves. Then add one or two other herbs (from the list on pp.97–9), which you feel may be therapeutic. Add a few drops of vegetable oil and tie up the bag with ribbon or twine. Place it underneath your main pillow. Refill your herbal pillow regularly.

claim that hops induce sleep more rapidly than valerian (see opposite). Hops should not be taken if you are depressed.

JAMAICAN DOGWOOD

The bark of this tree, which grows in the Caribbean, in Mexico and in Texas, is dried for use in liquid extracts and powders. A strong remedy for sleeplessness, it should not be taken if you are pregnant, or suffer from heart problems. It should only be used according to the instructions of a qualified practitioner.

LADY'S SLIPPER

Used by Native North Americans as tranquillizers, the roots of this plant treat sleeplessness associated with stress, emotional tension and anxiety. The rhizomes, or roots, are dried and made into infusions, liquid extracts and powders.

LAVENDER

The flowers are reputed to have anti-depressant and anti-spasmodic effects. Herbal literature suggests that lavender is

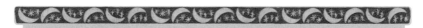

THE BALM OF LAVENDER

One of the main aromatherapy oils used in the promotion of sleep is lavender. There are many ways in which you can use this oil. Try inhaling its vapours, or mixing it with another oil, such as neroli, and massaging your partner. Or add the mixture to your bath. Alternatively, soak a cloth in warm water containing a few drops of lavender oil and place it across your forehead.

particularly beneficial in improving the sleep of people who are suffering from depression, while conventional wisdom indicates that it particularly helps sleeplessness in the elderly. The oil can be added to baths or used in aromatherapy massages.

PEPPERMINT

This herb is used as a digestive aid, decongestant, anesthetic and germicide; it has also been approved by the US Food and Drug Administration as a remedy for the common cold. Peppermint is said to promote relief from many of the symptoms that may interfere with normal sleep. It is helpful for spasms and headaches, and is used to treat nervousness, insomnia and dizziness. It is taken as a herbal tea.

ROMAN CAMOMILE

Used primarily for their anti-spasmodic and anti-inflammatory properties, the flowers of this plant are made into a herbal tea to make a gentle sedative that can help relieve anxiety and insomnia.

VALERIAN

Valerian is recognized as a sedative in both alternative and conventional medicine. The roots of the plant are used in infusions to treat insomnia. Commercially-manufactured tablets are also available. It is one of the few herbs that has been tested by recognized scientific techniques. Research has shown that valerian can improve sleep without leaving the patient with the usual "hangover" associated with sleep medications, such as sleeping pills. Interestingly, one study found that this herb helped smokers to sleep more soundly. Research supports herbalists' recommendations to use valerian to treat insomnia, nervousness, anxiety, headaches and intestinal cramps.

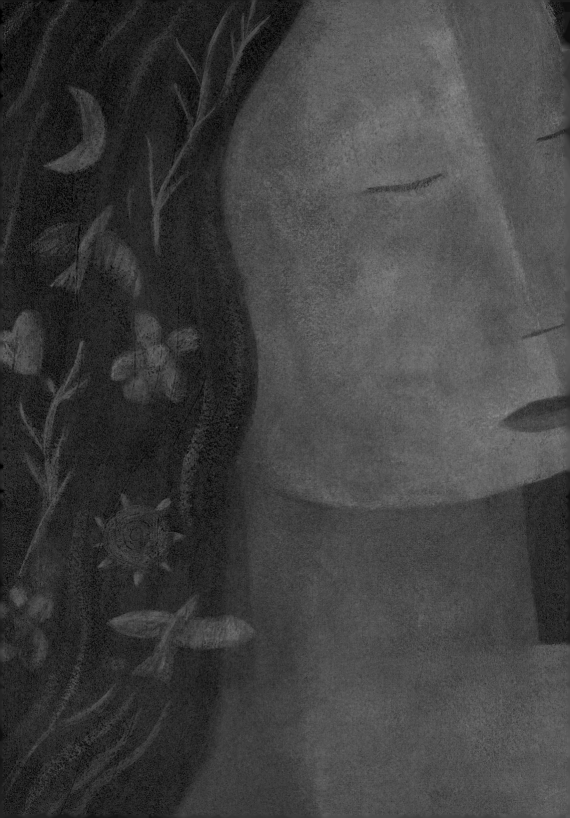

A Mind for Sleep

If the brain is the organ in which our thought processes take place, the mind is surely the consciousness that gives our thoughts context and meaning. As we have seen, some sleep difficulties stem from the way in which our brain regulates various physical cycles over which we have no voluntary control, such as the biological clock. But other disturbances happen as a result of mental activity that we knowingly generate, such as worrying, and such problems can often be tackled directly by learning how to relax our mind and banish the noise of mental chatter.

In this chapter, we explore ways to prepare our mind for refreshing sleep, gaining inspiration from techniques both ancient and modern. Some of these methods — for example, meditation — are drawn from the spiritual path to enlightenment followed in Buddhism, Hinduism and other Eastern religions; while others, such as the more recent techniques of visualization and hypnotherapy, harness the imagination and the creative powers of the mind to help us improve the quality of our sleep.

Banishing Worries

When we cannot sleep, physical or, more often, mental discomfort is usually to blame. We tell ourselves: "I can't switch off," "I wake up and my mind is racing," "I can't stop thinking about x,y,z," "I'm worried about not sleeping and what it will do to me," and so the list goes on. One of the best methods for dealing with a lack of sleep caused by worry is to learn "thought management". Expelling those obsessive, anxiety-inducing, wakefulness-promoting thoughts from our mind can be the key to good sleep. So how do we prevent ourselves from wishing we could change past situations that still make us feel angry or embarrassed? Or from lying awake, dreading future events?

A good starting point is to try to put our anxieties regarding the past into perspective. Some of us have a tendency to distort our view of life. Everything is either black or white – in any given situation we see ourselves either as a great success or as a miserable failure, when most situations in life can actually be defined in shades of grey. It is fine (and healthy) to set yourself high standards, and to try to analyze why, for example, you only achieved a Grade B in an examination when you expected to obtain a Grade A, but you also need to learn how to accept and acknowledge the validity of Grade B. One approach is to arm yourself with positive statements that disable the negative ones. For example, if you are constantly condemning yourself to failure by setting yourself perfectionist targets, before going to bed affirm to yourself: "It's OK to be less than perfect," or "No one is perfect," or "No one says I

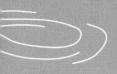

Exercise 11

THE BIRDS OF PEACE

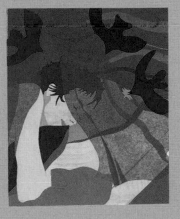

An inability to let go of anxiety when trying to sleep or after waking up during the night just leads to sleeplessness. Set aside approximately 30 minutes each evening specifically for dealing with your worries. It may help to write them down and to make a note of any action you can take the next day to resolve them. Then try the following exercise to banish them from your mind in preparation for sleep.

1. Sit somewhere comfortable and close your eyes. Turn your attention inward and focus on your breath. Inhale slowly and deeply until you start to relax.

2. Imagine yourself surrounded by a flock of black birds, which are flying around you, vying for your attention. The birds symbolize your anxieties — the biggest representing your most pressing concerns, and so on. Focus on the largest bird and the particular worry it embodies. As it swoops down toward you, catch it in your hands. Feel how light it is and ask yourself how something so insubstantial could weigh so heavily on your mind.

3. Now release the black bird and, with it, that particular worry. Watch as the bird flies away, changing from black to white as it soars into the sky.

4. Repeat this process with as many birds as you can, taking a few moments after you let each one go to enjoy the relief and peace that you experience.

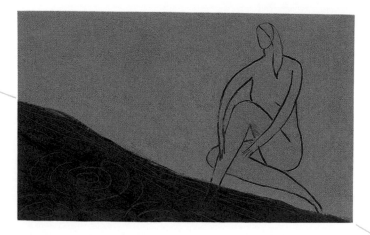

have to be perfect." If you repeat your chosen affirmation at least ten times each night, its message will slowly filter through to your unconscious. Once you start to accept the past, you will probably find that you acquire a new-found confidence in the future. But if you still find yourself constantly worrying that the worst will happen, use the same method, this time telling yourself: "Whether I worry or not, the outcome will be the same," or "Things often turn out better than I expect." The principle is the same: replace your pessimism with an optimistic message.

Another useful type of "thought management" is to try to analyze as objectively as possible whether your worries are justified or whether you have a distorted view of them. During sleepless nights, it is so easy to jump to negative conclusions that lack any supporting evidence — for example, by focusing completely on any bad or unfavourable aspects of a situation and totally disregarding or denying the good aspects. Or perhaps you believe that because you *feel* you are a failure in one respect, you will automatically fail at anything you try. If this sounds like the type of reasoning you are guilty of when you cannot sleep, try the following technique to help you put your worries into perspective.

Let us assume you have recently been interviewed for a new job and that you are awaiting notification of the outcome. In the meantime your sleep has been adversely affected: you keep waking up in the night and replaying the interview over and over in your mind. You feel that you performed badly and do not expect to be offered the job. Now cast your mind back to the interview and imagine that you are the interviewer. Replay the interaction exactly as you remember it, but this time envisage your performance from the perspective of a reasonable and experienced interviewer. For example, while you might feel that asking about pay reviews and bonuses made you appear mercenary, the interviewer may have felt that such questions showed that you value yourself and your skills and expect to be paid well for them.

When you do an exercise such as this, it can help to write down your findings, so that you can weigh up the "evidence" that both supports and contradicts any original assessment that you made. Make two columns and in one put your own impressions of the situation. In the other note down the impressions that the other person or people present might have gained, or how they might have felt about the situation. Once you have gathered the data, consider all the different interpretations, which may range from endorsing your viewpoint to totally contradicting it, and decide which is the most plausible. You may conclude that your instinct was right – things could have gone better – but you may also realize that an interaction or experience was not nearly as bad as you first thought. At the very least, assessing and analyzing your worries in this way can enable you to see them more dispassionately. This in turn can help you fight your tendency to distort reality and make sleep-disrupting worry a thing of the past.

Casting Off Anger

Anger is a stress response which involves both the body and the mind. If we have angry thoughts, our body reacts accordingly: epinephrine (adrenaline) is released, our heart rate goes up, and our muscles become tense. We are primed, ready for action. This state of arousal is exactly the antithesis of the state required for sleep. It is therefore vitally important to deal with anger before we go to bed, as otherwise we will be too agitated to sleep.

One way to improve sleep is to ensure that we have a regular outlet for our aggression. Pent-up anger can give rise to major sleep disruption, and by causing deficits in our sleep this powerful emotion can make us irritable and aggressive, thus building up a vicious circle. How, then, should you try to release your anger? There are many different approaches. You could do something physical and take up a competitive sport, such as squash or tennis, go for workouts at the gym or learn the grace and discipline of a martial art such as T'ai Chi (see pp.88–9). Or perhaps you would benefit more from practising a gentler form of release, such as yoga, meditation or visualization techniques. Any of these disciplines will both work off your pent-up anger and generally benefit your health, as well as, of course, improving your sleep.

As a rule, it is best to avoid arguments and confrontations as bedtime draws near. But if you suddenly find yourself in such a situation, what should you do? You may be able to cast off your anger by writing down your feelings on paper and then tearing them up. However, if all else fails, it may help to let off steam by punching a pillow in one quick burst of raw emotion.

Exercise 12

LETTING GO

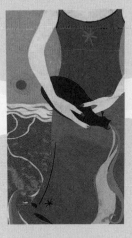

If you find yourself in a situation where the intensity of your anger over a particular matter is keeping you awake, try this exercise to help you dissipate your angry feelings and release tension.

1. Find a small, hard object, such as a large coin or a pebble. Sit somewhere comfortable and squeeze the object as hard as you can in the palm of your hand, while at the same time counting to 10 (you will probably find that you hold your breath as you do this). Exhale and release the object, this time counting to five. Repeat the squeezing and releasing movements three times.

2. Keeping the object in your hand, empty your mind and focus on your breath — inhaling and exhaling slowly, deeply and rhythmically for approximately five minutes. If you find unwanted thoughts creeping into your mind, try to observe them in a detached manner — acknowledge their existence but let them come and go without reacting to them.

3. Gently reflect on your feelings. Acknowledge that you have a right to be annoyed, but try to accept that undesirable events and behaviour are part of life, and resolve to deal with your negative feelings constructively. Open your hand and stroke the coin or pebble, then put it away in a drawer or cupboard. You have let go of your anger. You are once more at peace with yourself.

The Power of Meditation

Meditation, the process of consciously stilling the body and especially the mind to promote deep relaxation, has been practised in the East for thousands of years. As improving our sleep relies heavily upon developing our ability to relax when we are awake, it is worth spending a little while here exploring the practice of meditation.

From a scientific point of view, the brain waves experienced during deep meditation are similar to those of light sleep – alpha waves are characteristic of both. Although we have to be well-practised in meditation to reach such a state, there are many benefits to be gained, even at the beginner's level. Meditation is sometimes referred to as "restful alertness", an apparently contradictory, but actually true definition, because the state of meditation marries the physical attributes of sleep with those of wakefulness. During sleep our heart rate lowers, our metabolism becomes slower, we consume less oxygen and our conscious awareness of the outside world disappears. All these things are true of meditation too – except that, although we seem to have little conscious awareness of the outside world while we practise, we are, in fact, mentally fully alert throughout. And at a very advanced level, *yogis* are said to be able to meditate instead of sleeping – however, I would not recommend that you try this!

You can make a start upon improving your sleep by incorporating meditation into your regular bedtime routine. The exercise on the opposite page takes you step by step through a pre-sleep meditation – in this case the focus is the flicker of a candle flame, but you could use any

Exercise 13

A CANDLE-FLAME MEDITATION

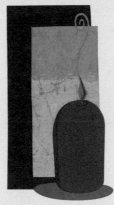

One of the most common causes of sleeplessness is an inability to "switch off" our racing mind. An effective way to train ourselves to do so is to use a pre-sleep, single-point meditation. This exercise guides you on how to focus your mind on a candle flame, whose endlessly varied flickering can promote deep relaxation.

1. Light the candle and, placing it safely, sit in a comfortable position in front of it. Relax your shoulders, and gaze into the flame. Soften your focus so that you are not staring at the flame but gazing as if to see through and beyond it.

2. Bring your attention to the corona around the flame. Notice how the edge of the flame distils into a gentle haze. Squint your eyes a little — notice how doing so causes shafts of light to seem to throw themselves from the flame, like the last, warm rays of the sun as it dips beneath the horizon at the end of the day. Make a connection in your mind between this image and thoughts of bedtime.

3. Now close your eyes and imagine the warm glow of the flame filling your consciousness. It is calm, safe and comforting. Breathe deeply for a few minutes, basking in your sense of inner tranquillity. (If your attention wanders, open your eyes and bring your focus back to the real flame, then close your eyes again.) Once you feel completely calm and your mind is empty, slowly open your eyes and gently blow out the candle. You feel relaxed and ready for bed.

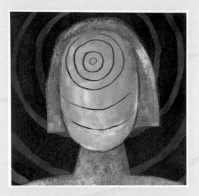

"sleepy" image. You need only spend ten or fifteen minutes each night meditating, but doing so will undoubtedly release the stress of the day and put you in mind for sleep.

However, before you try the exercise, bear in mind that it can be helpful to break meditation down into four separate stages, the first two of which are most relevant to helping you to sleep better. The first stage is *preparation* — most importantly the preparation of your environment. Choose somewhere quiet and tranquil. As this is a pre-sleep meditation, the ideal place would be your bedroom, as this will reinforce associations with peace and relaxation. It is also probably the most practical place, as it may well be the only room in the house in which you are likely to be left undisturbed. Try to ensure that the room is tidy — if you are emptying your mind of troubling thoughts, you need to make sure that your environment is free of clutter too. Although it may be tempting, try to resist the urge to meditate on your bed, which should be reserved for sleeping and sex only! Select a cushion or pillow which you can keep especially for your meditation practice and sit on this on the floor. Wear comfortable, loose clothing and choose a position that you can maintain effortlessly for an extended period of time (for example, you may decide to sit cross-legged, but there is certainly no need to try to push your-self into the Lotus position).

The second stage in meditation is *application*, in which we select the focus for our practice. When we first begin to meditate, it can help to focus the mind on something to stop distracting thoughts hijacking our concentration. The exercise on p.109 uses a candle flame, but your could try anything with connota-tions of sleep: for example, the moon, a feather (from your down quilt), even the letter "z"! Whatever you select, ensure that it does not have associations with your sleep problems – for example, focusing on a clockface showing your ideal bedtime might have the negative effect of reminding you how much later it usually is before you succeed in falling asleep. Once you have chosen the focus for your meditation, recreate it in your mind's eye in as much detail as possible. Hold the image there until all distracting thoughts are stilled, then gradually try to empty your mind by letting the image fade away. If you find this difficult and thoughts start to intrude, bring your mental image back into focus for a while before fading it out again.

The third and fourth stages of meditation, reached by advanced practitioners, are *realization* and *transformation*. In the former, the meditator witnesses the universal truth – that we exist in spirit form within our physical bodies, which are them-selves merely the vehicles of our existence and not the essence. Transformation is the act by which the *yogi* reaches *nirvana* – the final spiritual goal in which physical form is overcome by the enlightened spirit. When you meditate with the aim of promoting sleep, bear in mind that we are essentially spiritual beings who can rise above the baggage we carry in the material world, but do not become distracted by this philosophy – accept it as a truth.

Patterns of the Cosmos

Widely used in Eastern meditation, mandalas and yantras are visual representations of the universe that can be memorized and brought into the mind as a focus for the mind's eye. Mandalas range from a simple circle with a dot in the centre to highly complex, geometric images, sometimes partly figurative, that are full of religious or spiritual symbolism. Yantras on the other hand do not contain any human or animal likenesses — instead they symbolize the universe purely in geometric shapes. As an aid for getting a good night's sleep, the value of mandalas and yantras is to provide us with a focus for the mind in meditation. By distracting the mind from worries and alerting thoughts, these intriguing images can help us to relax into a state of tranquillity, and ultimately, sleep.

The Swiss psychoanalyst Carl Jung (1875–1961) noticed that some of his patients, who had no knowledge necessarily of Eastern mysticism, began to draw and paint mandala-like pictures. Jung became intrigued by the idea that mandalas and

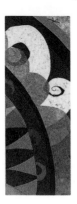

yantras are universal symbols from the "collective unconscious", representing the primal order of the psyche. It is certainly true that these patterns appear in all cultures. For example, they are present in such diverse forms as Native North American sand paintings, the rose windows of Christian churches, and in nature itself as snow crystals and many-petalled flowers. The exercise (opposite) shows you how to create your own mandalas or yantras and use them as a focus for pre-sleep meditation.

Exercise 14

CREATING YOUR OWN SLEEP MANDALA

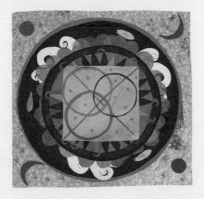

If you design your own mandala or yantra as a visual meditation to help you to sleep, whether consciously or unconsciously you are likely to create a pattern that is symbolically meaningful to you, and therefore easier to work with. When you have devised your mandala or yantra, sign and date it and put it somewhere where you can see it regularly, to help to fix it in your mind.

1. Take a large piece of paper and draw or paint a big circle in the middle. Add some other geometric shapes to form a pattern within the circle. Choose your colours carefully. Use predominantly relaxing shades, such as blues and greens, that are easy on the eye.

2. Fill the circle with whatever you feel belongs there, but remember that the purpose of the mandala is to help you improve your sleep and that your design should reflect this theme. For example, you could perhaps incorporate a closed eye, some stars or musical notes (to remind you of your favourite relaxing music) in your design.

3. To use your mandala as a meditation aid, place your design at eye level, at a comfortable distance from the place where you sit to meditate. Sit down on your cushion or pillow and close your eyes. Concentrate on your breathing for two minutes to still your body and mind. When you feel ready, open your eyes and focus on your mandala.

Visions of Sleep

Fundamental to all ancient meditative traditions is the act of visualization. When we practise a visualization, we watch in our mind's eye the scene, object, person or action in as much real-life detail as possible — the more vivid and lifelike the image, the more effective the visualization. The act of visualization is useful in the quest for sleep improvement for two reasons. First

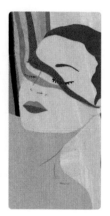

(and most specifically), it has the advantage of focusing our mind fully on matters other than any anxiety we might have about sleep; and second, as a form of meditation, it regulates our breathing, slowing our heart rate and encouraging relaxation.

One of the most effective uses for visualization in sleep improvement is as a sleep trigger. If we can create for ourselves the perfect sleeping place in our mind's eye, we can return to this place each time we wish to fall asleep. And the same technique can be used if we wake during the night and find it hard to return to sleep. First, think of the most relaxing place you can imagine. This might be somewhere that you have actually visited, such as a tranquil forest glade where you once spent a lazy summer afternoon; or somewhere that you imagine as the most restful place on earth, such as a secluded tropical beach. Close your eyes and breathe deeply for a few minutes. Try to empty your mind of distracting thoughts. Conjure up an image of the restful place. Visualize it in as much detail as you possibly can. Let us assume it is the forest glade. What trees surround you? Is the glade partly shaded or bathed in enveloping sunlight? What tones of green can you see in the leaves, the grass and the other foliage? Can you smell the damp soil? Do you hear birds singing? In your imagination think of this place in all its glorious detail. Visualize yourself lying peacefully in your restful place. Feel the comforting support of Mother Earth under your back. Now focus on one sound – if it is birdsong, imagine the tune lulling you into sleep just as your mother used to sing you lullabies. Feel the warmth of the sun on your skin – you are bathed in the rays of its goodness. Breathe deeply and with each breath imagine drifting further and further into sleep. Now you are gone ...

HONING YOUR OBSERVATION SKILLS

*

One of the keys to establishing a successful pre-sleep visualization lies in honing your general powers of observation. Start simply. When you eat, regard your meal as a feast for your eyes as well as your palate. Absorb all the colours of the food on your plate and concentrate on the various tastes as you chew (effective visualization is enormously enhanced if we can employ all our senses to conjure up an image). On your walk to work pay attention to the buildings you see – what is each used for? Are there any interesting "landmarks" such as an antique mailbox, a newspaper stand or a flower stall? Can you identify the trees along the sidewalk or the flowers growing on the verges? Do you know the names of all the streets on your route? You may be surprised at how much detail usually passes you by as you hurry along every morning, lost in your own inner world. By developing your powers of observation in this way you will be able to make your pre-sleep visualization more vivid and plausible.

The Power of Suggestion

The ancient Egyptians and Greeks are said to have put patients into a trance to promote healing, while African and American tribal cultures have long used drumming and dancing for hypnotic effect. Since its discovery by the Austrian physician Franz Anton Mesmer in the late eighteenth century, hypnosis has been used by generations of doctors and psychotherapists in the West to encourage patients to cure themselves by implanting in their minds a suggestion that they are able to do so.

When James Braid embarked on the first scientific investigation of hypnosis in the nineteenth century, he pronounced it to be a form of "nervous sleep", similar to natural sleep but induced by the patient's concentration on the hypnotist. However, more recent research shows that the brain waves of hypnotized subjects closely resemble those of people who are awake.

Contemporary hypnotherapy involves putting the patient into a deeply relaxed state in which their critical faculties are suspended. The hypnotherapist can then implant positive suggestions into the subconscious mind that will affect the perception or behaviour of the person both during and after the trance.

Hypnotherapy has proved that it can successfully treat some of the common causes of insomnia, such as pain and anxiety. While there is little research to indicate whether hypnotism can improve sleep directly, it may be worth trying the direct approach, in which the hypnotist may suggest, for example, that your hot, milky bedtime drink is actually a powerful sleeping potion, which will make you fall asleep as soon as you go to bed and give you eight hours of refreshing, quality sleep.

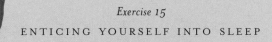

Exercise 15

ENTICING YOURSELF INTO SLEEP

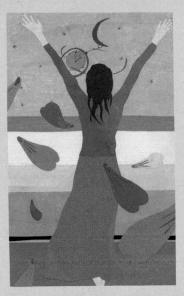

If you cannot visit a hypnotherapist, try the following exercise in self-hypnosis to improve your sleep. (Note: anyone with mental problems should seek medical advice before trying self-hypnosis.)

1. Lie on the floor in a comfortable position, your arms by your sides. Focus on your breathing, feeling yourself sink into the floor as you completely relax.

2. Fix your gaze on a point on the ceiling and take five, progressively longer breaths. As you exhale each time, tell yourself: "I am ready to go to sleep."

3. Imagine yourself going down 10 stairs into a beautiful bedroom. As you descend, count down from 10 to one, and try to feel increasingly relaxed. Watch yourself lie down on the sumptuous bed and sink into the soft covers. Tell yourself, "I am falling deeply asleep," as in your mind's eye you drift off. Focus on your sleeping figure and breathe deeply.

4. Tell yourself: "On the count of three, I will wake up feeling totally relaxed and ready for sleep." Count to three. Slowly get up and go straight to bed.

Sounds Asleep

During early sleep research experiments, subjects were asked to sleep in anechoic (echoless) rooms. Although we might think that silence is the optimum aural environment for sleep, the researchers actually found that it had an adverse effect on the sleep of their subjects. Looked at closely, the conclusions of that early research seem perfectly logical. We are enveloped by sound at all stages of our existence. In the womb, hearing is one of the earliest senses to develop, and as we grow we are soothed by the sounds of the amniotic fluid and our mother's voice. As

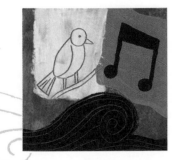

adults, even when we take a few moments to relish what we call "silence", what we really mean is that we have temporarily escaped being disrupted by noise. But undoubtedly some noise is still present – the echo of a child's voice, the hum of passing traffic, the natural sound of birdsong.

So although we might think that we should soundproof our bedrooms, what we really need to do is to free ourselves from disruptive and disturbing noise. Of course there are practical solutions, such as mending a broken door latch that clatters, but other annoying noises – for example, a neighbour's dog barking or a party in the same apartment block – can be difficult to stop as they are beyond our immediate control. In these cases (and if we have difficulty sleeping anyway), providing our own sleep-promoting sounds can be invaluable, whether to muffle the noise that disturbs us, or to provide another focus for the mind, or simply to trigger the mood of sleep.

We all have our own ideas about which sounds we find most relaxing, but one of the most accessible and universally enjoyable is music. If you like listening to music, why not keep a special selection for pre-bedtime listening, and try to incorporate half an hour's listening into your normal pre-sleep routine? Better still, if you have a cassette-tape player, you can record your own sequence of tracks, compiling a series of tunes or pieces that are increasingly relaxing – gentle melodies can caress our senses and ease away physical tension. Find somewhere comfortable, perhaps the couch in the living room, and just sit back and listen. (Although it may be tempting to lie on your bed, some believe that this is not a good idea – in Feng Shui, for example, the radiation emitted from electrical equipment is believed to cause an imbalance of energy in your bedroom and so impair your sleep.)

Everyone is used to having music in the background, but if you are using music to help you prepare for sleep, try actively to engage with it. Immerse yourself in the music, bringing it to the foreground. Experiment with different combinations of pieces until you discover your own perfect pre-sleep selection.

ROCK-A-BYE BABY

*

Few of us realize that babies in the womb are already sensitive to sound. Recent experiments have shown that if an unborn child regularly hears the same song during pregnancy, he or she will come to associate it with the security of the womb. Then, when the infant is exposed to the same song after he or she is born, the familiar sounds will be comforting and help to encourage sleep.

Routines and Rituals

While novelty wakes the brain up — and also generates stress hormones — routines tend to settle it down. Sleep is partly a learned behaviour, and so the conditions we come to associate with going to sleep ultimately help us to drift off. Routines provide a basis for developing such associations.

It is up to each of us individually to decide how soon before sleep we embark upon a bedtime routine. For most of us this is an automatic, almost robotic period, in which we go through the ritual of washing, cleaning our teeth, changing for bed, getting into bed and then perhaps reading a few chapters of a book. Prayer might also be part of the routine. Then, when we finally turn off the light, we expect that our brain will recognize this as the time for mental shut-down and relax into sleep.

However, for most of us getting off to sleep is rarely that simple. Many of us have a problem switching off our minds and sometimes we need to re-learn the primary association that we learned as a baby — that bed is a place for sleeping, not thinking. One way to reinforce this attitude is to set aside a short period of time before attempting to fall asleep, to make a conscious effort to deal with unfinished business. First, this means not reading in bed! Although we may find it a relaxing pastime because it forces

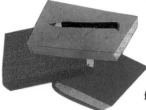

our mind to think about something other than the anxieties of the day, reading engages our attention, and disengages our mind from the purpose of sleep. The bed is not a place for concentration — it is for sleep and (apart from sex) only sleep!

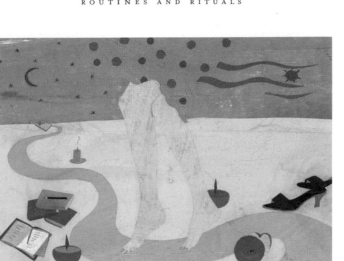

A bedtime ritual, therefore, must consist of activities that consciously empty your mind to prepare you for bed. First, note down any issues that are concerning you on a piece of paper, then fold up the paper and set it aside for the next day and banish the issues from your mind — anything that you wrote down is better dealt with after a refreshing night's sleep. Get yourself ready for bed, and try to empty your mind of meandering thoughts using a meditation or visualization (any of the ones in this book will do). If any thoughts creep in, let them simply pass through your head, without allowing them to settle. Only once you feel ready for sleep should you get into bed.

Of course, it is not only adults who need bedtime routines. Children, too, often find it hard to settle down at night and can find it comforting to have a nightly ritual. Establish a predictable routine — for example, a bath or shower, followed by dressing for bed and then half an hour doing any restful activity that will help them to settle. Do not be tempted to bend the rules — at the end of the half-hour, it is time for bed!

The Nature of Dreams

This may seem an unusual idea, but we have within our grasp the opportunity to improve sleep *using* sleep. As we already know, REM sleep is also known as dreaming sleep, but the difference between REM sleep and dreaming itself is similar to the distinction between the physical properties of the brain and the consciousness we experience with our mind. In other words, our brain activity can be measured and viewed objectively, whereas our dreams are unique, highly subjective and unquantifiable mental events. These events are believed by many to present opportunities for greater understanding of our unconscious, and through that understanding we can achieve increased self-knowledge and overall wellbeing. In addition, we already know

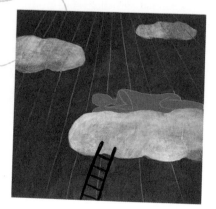

that dreaming sleep comes second in the hierarchy of important stages of sleep, so by encouraging our dreams and learning from them we not only improve our self-understanding, but also maximize this fundamental aspect of our sleeping pattern.

Dreaming has intrigued the human race since time immemorial, but Sigmund Freud (1856–1939), the famous Viennese psychiatrist, was the first scientist who expressly declared that he considered dreams to be the "royal road to the unconscious" — a means of accessing the non-conscious parts of the mind. (Freud's contemporary, the Swiss Carl Jung, on the other hand, formulated the idea that some dreams are an expression of the reservoir of racial memories and experiences that are possessed by every one of us. He termed this storehouse of knowledge the *collective unconscious*.)

During the 1990s, Ernest Hartmann of Tufts University, Boston, using data derived primarily from dreams recalled by trauma victims, argued that the main function of dreaming is to calm the mind, which is bombarded, and consequently overloaded, with stimuli during waking hours. He suggests that during dreaming, deep cross-connections (which are not made during wakefulness) are formed in the brain, thereby dissipating energy and allowing the brain to "let off steam". By increasing the number of cross-associations that are created in the brain, this process may have the added advantage of aiding the consolidation of memory. The release of energy in the brain may

THE DREAM CATCHERS

One of the customs of the Ojibwe, a Native North American people, is to place hoops known as "dreamcatchers" next to their babies' cradle boards to protect them from bad dreams. The dreamcatchers derive from an ancient myth about Asibikasshi (Spider Woman), a sun deity, who spun webs around the sleeping places of babies to filter out bad dreams. When the tribes scattered, Asibikasshi was unable to reach all the children so the women began weaving their own dreamcatchers. They used willow hoops, whose circular shape represents the sun, criss-crossed with "string" made from plant fibres. The web is attached to the hoop at eight points, representing Asibikasshi's legs, and there is a small central hole to allow the good dreams through.

also trigger the mind to represent our dominant waking emotions and concerns metaphorically in our dreams. For example, the fear and terror experienced by the trauma victims was expressed by dreams as events such as "running from a huge tidal wave".

The work of Freud, Jung and Hartmann forms the basis of techniques employed by many psychotherapists and psycho-analysts in stress management (part of which includes sleep improvement) today. If we explore the messages from our unconscious conveyed in our dreams, we can achieve greater self-understanding, which can give us the strength to tackle any problems in our waking life that are adversely affecting our sleep. The exercise opposite presents a way to encourage vivid recollec-tion of your dreams.

But what of using dream cues? Through this technique many people are able to promote dreams on specific problems in their waking lives to try to find solutions from their unconscious. To cue your dreams to focus on improving your sleep, meditate for a few moments on an image that, for you, embodies deep relax-ation or refreshing sleep. For example, perhaps you imagine yourself relaxing peacefully in your garden, in the shade of an apple tree, on a warm summer's afternoon. Hold this scene in your mind for a few moments, visualizing it in as much detail as possible. Can you feel the gentle breeze caressing your body? What is the sweet scent you smell? Note how sleepy and content you feel. Hold this image of perfect tranquillity in your mind and tell yourself that this is how you wish to feel every night as you drift off. With any luck this exercise will guide you safe-ly into dreaming sleep, where your unconscious mind can perhaps suggest other ways to improve your rest.

Exercise 16

HOW TO RECALL YOUR DREAMS

Most of us remember only brief fragments of our dreams, but it is possible to learn how to recall them in more detail. Try this exercise every night for a week – it will help you to discover any important, recurrent themes.

1. Before retiring, place a pencil and paper within easy reach of your bed. Reflect on any topics that were often in your thoughts during the day.

2. As you settle down to sleep, relax and clear your mind of mental clutter, allowing thoughts to drift across your mind without paying them any attention and letting sleep come naturally.

3. If you awaken during the night, write down any dreams you have had in as much detail as possible. You can make a sketch instead, if this makes it easier to express the content of your dream.

4. When you wake up in the morning, write down any dreams that you can remember, noting key emotions as well as people, places, events and so on.

5. Analyze your dream report to see if any particular themes emerge.

6. Compare the content of your dreams with the topics that were often in your thoughts the day before, noting any obvious links, coincidences, symbols and so on. You may be surprised by the associations you find.

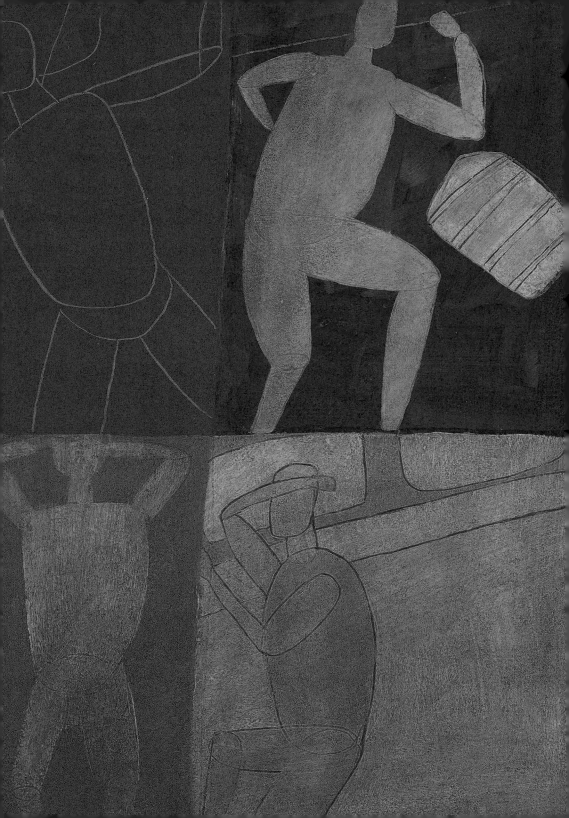

Overcoming Sleep Problems

Many of the techniques described so far will help promote natural sleep for those of us whose sleep simply needs some improvement. However, there are others of us whose sleep is more drastically affected by a "sleep disorder" – a clinically diagnosable condition that prevents us from sleeping properly. It can be many years before a sleep disorder is diagnosed – mainly because there are so many emotional or environmental factors that impair our sleep, and doctors rarely have time to work through all the possibilities with their patients. However, sleep disorders are serious and extremely debilitating conditions so, to help you recognize the tell-tale signs, over the following pages we look at some of the most common disorders, such as insomnia, sleepwalking, nightmares and the more dangerous sleep apnea, among others, and offer some practical advice on how to cope with them and where possible how to use self-help techniques to relieve their symptoms. We also take a look at insomnia caused by jetlag and shift work, and we conclude with practical tips on what to do when our partner's troubled sleep keeps us awake at night.

Defining and Tackling Insomnia

Before we can begin to think about overcoming insomnia, it is crucial that we understand exactly what it is. The dictionary definition of the disorder calls it a "prolonged inability to sleep", but even this only scratches the surface.

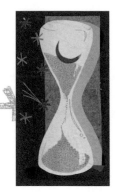

Crucially, we must remember that sleeplessness and insomnia are not the same thing. Sleeplessness describes a condition that nearly everyone understands: a period of time when someone desires sleep but does not get it. This can occur during the day or night – for example, if someone tries to have a nap in the afternoon and is unable to go to sleep, or if a parent goes to bed and a young child wakes them up and subsequently the parent cannot get back to sleep. Insomnia, on the other hand, is a condition that occurs when someone who has previously been a good sleeper suffers from chronic (lasting several weeks at least) sleeplessness.

Three types of insomnia have been identified: *psychophysiological insomnia*; *idiopathic insomnia*; and *sleep-state misperception*. The most common of these, **psychophysiological insomnia** (also known as conditioned or learned insomnia), is usually triggered by a life event such as bereavement or losing a job. The Bootzin Stimulus Control procedure (see box, opposite) can help sufferers overcome the disorder – particularly if they can deal with the underlying problem at the same time. For example, if an insomniac starts worrying about their sleep, the anxiety caused by the worry may further exacerbate the insomnia, so the condition worsens. Relaxation techniques, including breathing, meditation, massage and aromatherapy — all of which are covered in this book — can help to break the cycle of worrying about poor sleep (which itself causes even poorer sleep) by relieving the psychological pressure and so helping to ease the body into sleep. Additionally, try rearranging your bedroom or even moving your bed to another room in the house. Conditioned insomniacs characteristically associate the bed, and sometimes the room, with sleeplessness, so changing the room in some way can help to relieve another psychological block to sleep.

Idiopathic insomnia, also known as childhood onset insomnia, is a lifelong condition. Sufferers of this disorder tend to be in good general health and there is no obvious life event that could have acted as a trigger. Abnormal EEG readings in the sleep state have led scientists to believe that idiopathic insomnia is caused because the sleep–wake centres in the brain (see pp.32–3) do not work properly. This condition is understandably difficult to cure. Optimizing the conditions for sleep

THE BOOTZIN STIMULUS CONTROL

American sleep expert Richard Bootzin has developed a comprehensive technique for tackling conditioned insomnia. The following steps should help insomniacs aged between 20 and 60.

• Go to bed only when you feel sleepy • Keep your bed as a place for sleep and sex only • If you do not fall asleep within 20 minutes, get out of bed and do something else • Return to bed once you feel sleepy (and get up again if necessary) • Set your alarm to wake you up at the same time every day — and do not sleep in • Do not nap during the day.

through the usual techniques (looking at environment and physical and mental wellbeing) are important but, currently, idiopathic insomniacs require pharmacological help to get to sleep.

The third type of insomnia, **sleep-state misperception**, is diagnosed when EEG readings show that someone seems to be asleep, but the person subsequently claims that they were awake. Very little is known about this type of insomnia, and indeed it is often not recognized as a sleep disorder at all. For those who suffer from it, the condition is highly debilitating. If you are a sufferer, first look at why you believe you have not slept. Is it that you have very vivid and lifelike dreams? Before you go to bed, try a visualization (which may also help sufferers of psychophysiological insomnia). Prepare yourself for bed and then sit comfortably on the floor near your bed. Close your eyes and tense and relax each muscle group in turn, beginning with your feet and moving up your body. Imagine that as you "free" your muscles, you are bathed in white light, which makes you feel safe and warm. Once you have envisaged your whole body cocooned in this light for a few moments, open your eyes and get into bed, while retaining in your mind the image of yourself bathed in the light. Over time, you will drift into deep, restorative sleep.

When trying to break the cycle of any type of insomnia, keeping a journal (see pp.24–5) is crucial for pinpointing biological and psychological factors that might exacerbate the insomnia and offering encouragement by revealing even small improvements to your sleep. Once you have started using a journal regularly, the next step is to go back to basics. Set regular times to go to bed and to get up. Avoid alcohol, tobacco and caffeine, and do not exercise within three hours of bedtime. Also, ensure that the bedroom is light-proof and that your bed is conducive to restful sleep (see pp.54–7).

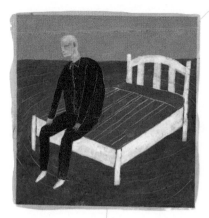

INSOMNIA AND DEPRESSION

Before leaving the subject of insomnia, it is important to mention its links with depression. Nowadays, many patients who visit their doctor complaining of sleeping problems are prescribed antidepressants, probably for two reasons: first, there is a reluctance among doctors to prescribe sleeping pills because of the risk of patient dependency; and second, doctors are taught that insomnia is associated with depression (and consultation time is usually too short for a full exploration of possible causes).

However, the links between the two are not straightforward. When we are not depressed, sleep disruption makes us feel low; but, if we are depressed, sleep deprivation can actually improve our mood! Studies have suggested that REM is the stage of sleep that is most implicated in the biological cause of depression. Deliberate sleep shortening, allowing say four hours' sleep a night, has an antidepressant effect, probably because it reduces the amount of early morning REM sleep that the sleeper gains. It may be, then, that when we are depressed we suffer from insomnia because the brain shortens the time devoted to dreaming sleep in an attempt to combat the depression.

The Nighttime Marathon

We have all experienced the sensation of needing to *do* something — even if we otherwise feel exhausted. Restlessness can come upon us at any time and it has no scientific explanation. It can manifest itself in bed in a surprisingly common syndrome known as *Restless Legs*. In this sleep disorder a strange, unpleasant creepy-crawly sensation is felt in the legs, which prevents the sufferer from going to sleep and forces them to get out of bed and walk around. Between three and eight per cent of the American population suffer from Restless Legs, and the figure rises to as many

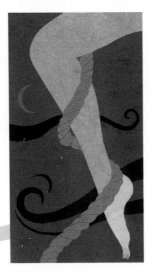

as thirty per cent among people suffering from rheumatoid arthritis. Fifteen per cent of women experience them in the last few months of pregnancy, although happily the condition usually disappears after they give birth.

Of course, Restless Legs is completely harmless in itself, but as it can cause sleeplessness, and even insomnia, its knock-on effects can be debilitating. If you suffer from Restless Legs try massaging your muscles two to three hours before you go to bed through gentle rubbing. Using both hands together, "stroke" each leg in turn. Although there is no scientific proof that massaging prior to sleep prevents the syndrome, massage does help to stimulate the release of built-up tension in the muscles, thus promoting relaxation and stillness.

Unfortunately, eighty per cent of individuals afflicted by Restless Legs also suffer from *Periodic Limb Movement Syndrome* (PLMS). In PLMS the limbs, usually the legs, twitch every thirty seconds or so. PLMS disturbs our sleep but usually without waking us. However, the disruption to our sleep is usually sufficient to make us feel the next day as if we have run a marathon! Even worse, it might cause sleep disturbance for our bed partner.

Doctors have been unable to pinpoint the causes of Restless Legs and PLMS (which can also occur in isolation). Lack of iron and too much tea or coffee have both been identified as possible causes, as well as a deficiency in calcium.

Finally, Restless Legs and PLMS should not be confused with "nocturnal leg cramps" (sometimes called Charley-horse). These are painful sensations of muscular tightness in the calf or foot which last for a few seconds and disappear spontaneously.

CONTROLLING RESTLESS LEGS

There are no hard-and-fast rules for overcoming Restless Legs and PLMS, but by following a few simple guidelines we should be able to minimize their effects and prevent them from resulting in insomnia. First, check your caffeine intake — there is a very strong correlation between caffeine and Restless Legs, possibly because caffeine slows down our absorption of iron. Second, reduce your alcohol intake. Third, exercise regularly and keep a diary to track both the exercise and the condition. Avoid exercising within three hours of bedtime. Finally, Restless Legs occurs mainly in the late evening and early night. If possible, delay your bedtime until well after midnight and sleep on until 9 or 10am.

The Terrors of Deep Sleep

In the nineteenth century, Dr John Polidori, an Edinburgh physician, wrote his medical thesis on *sleepwalking*, which is probably the most common disorder of deep sleep. Curiously, he had been among the group of literati in Geneva in 1816 which included the writers Mary Shelley and Lord Byron, who subsequently spent that summer writing ghost stories – most famously, *Frankenstein* (Shelley). Polidori correctly observed that anything that clouded the mind, such as alcohol or sleeping with our feet higher than our head, would increase the frequency of sleepwalking. However, his remedies – arming servants with whips to awaken the sleepwalker, or surrounding the bed with baths of ice-cold water – are not now recommended!

Sleepwalking can involve prolonged and quite complicated acts (there are some incredible stories of people who have got up, got dressed, got into the car and then driven for a hundred miles or so before waking up!). The condition is most common in children – probably because of their developing brain. Most amazingly, perhaps, the sleepwalker has absolutely no recollection that they ever left their bed, and it can be extremely difficult to wake them, although there is no danger in trying.

There is actually very little that can be done to prevent sleepwalking, so the only course of action is to ensure that the sleepwalker cannot harm themselves. Remove any objects that the sleepwalker could trip over; and if they have a phobia about, say, spiders, try placing plastic imitations at the exit to the bedroom to deter the walker from strolling too far. Although this sounds farfetched, it is a technique that has proved successful!

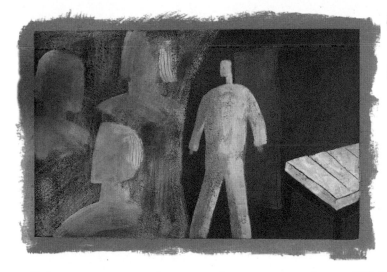

Night terrors are not *nightmares*: nightmares occur during REM, while night terrors are a feature of deep sleep. For some reason, the brain centres involved in controlling the expression of fear switch on without waking the person up. Night terrors often start with a piercing scream accompanied by the physical signs of fear: rapid heart-rate and breathing, perspiring and dilated pupils.

As with sleepwalking, night terrors occur mainly in children, although a small percentage of adults tends to suffer too. Importantly, we should remember that the condition carries no mental or physical health consequences – if you are a parent and your child suffers from them, the experience will probably worry you more than your child (who is unlikely to have any memory of the terror occurring). There are no certain ways to prevent night terrors, but you could try reducing the intensity of deep sleep by sleeping for longer. A nap in the late afternoon will also help "lighten" your nighttime sleep. It can take up to half an hour for a sufferer to awaken from a night terror – the best course of action for a parent or a partner is simply to keep them company through the experience.

The Terrors of Dreaming Sleep

As we have already seen, during the night we experience increasingly frequent and prolonged phases of dreaming sleep. We also know that we can use our dreams to improve our well-being and so our sleep. But what happens when our dreams are the cause of our sleeplessness? How do we cope with nightmares?

Nightmares occur mostly in pre-adolescent children, although, as with sleepwalking and night terrors, a small percentage of adults also frequently suffer from distressing dreams. Such dreams are often long and complicated, and they become increasingly frightening. The dreamer will wake up, usually fully alert, during the REM phase and will vividly recall the nightmare.

Periods of stress, trauma and some common medication (such as "beta-blockers", used to control blood pressure and panic attacks) promote nightmares. Some researchers believe that nightmares are the product of *sleep apnea* (see pp.146–9) – we begin to panic as we sleep because we feel that we cannot breathe, and this causes frightening visions in our dreams of such things as entrapment. However, more often than not, a nightmare is triggered by some emotional baggage deep within. In this respect we might consider the dreams as urgent messages from our

unconscious, drawing our attention to aspects of our inner self that demand our attention. Although nightmares are generally harmless, they can be so alarming as to make the sufferer fear sleep altogether. The exercise on the opposite page offers a technique for disarming this frightening aspect of sleep.

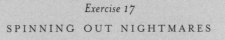

Exercise 17

SPINNING OUT NIGHTMARES

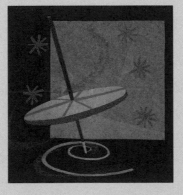

To confront the fears that appear in a nightmare, we can learn to extend the dream and overcome the experience. For this to happen, the nightmare needs to be "lucid" (we need to be aware that we are dreaming so that we can interact with the dream). Then, using the Spinning Technique invented by S. La Berge, we can disarm the nightmare.

1. Before you go to bed, sit quietly and tell yourself that you will be fully focused on your dreams. While you are dreaming, try to study the objects, actions and landscapes of your dreamworld. How are they bizarre or unreal? Mastering this technique can help to promote lucidity.

2. Once you are lucid, you can extend your dream beyond the point when you normally wake up. Start "spinning". Stretch out your dream arms and spin round like a top, moving freely over your dream landscape. While you spin tell yourself that the next thing you see, hear, touch or smell will be your nightmare.

3. Once you are in the nightmare, confront your fear. Engage in a dialogue with it (even if it is inanimately represented — say, as a tidal wave that might drown you or as walls that close in). Ask your fear why it appears in your dreams. Imagine it transforming into a friendlier image — a threatening stranger becomes a protective friend; a wave turns into lapping water on the seashore; walls fall away to reveal a serene landscape. Once you have transformed the image, come out of the dream. The nightmare is less likely to appear again.

Sleep Paralysis and Narcolepsy

Paralysis of the body's muscles occurs every night during REM sleep and is perfectly normal (see pp.42–3). Occasionally – once in a lifetime for nearly half of us – wakefulness occurs before the paralysis abates. This incredibly frightening experience means that for between one and two minutes after we wake up we are completely unable to move. Sleep paralysis renders the sufferer so still that many people during Victorian times left instructions in their wills that their wrists be cut before burial so that they were not accidentally buried alive (should the condition have been mistaken for death)!

Although the experience is frightening, there is in truth nothing dangerous about sleep paralysis at all. However, it can cause people to fear falling asleep. The condition tends to be hereditary and there are no obvious cures for it, so we must simply bear in mind that it will probably happen to us no more than once in a lifetime (if at all), and that if it does, the paralysis is certainly not permanent.

Just as there are no cures for sleep paralysis, there are also no obvious triggers. However, there is one section of any population that is more prone to the condition than any other. These are people who suffer from a syndrome called *narcolepsy*. Rather than being unable to sleep, narcoleptics are afflicted by sudden and uncontrollable bouts of sleep – often preceded by a complete loss of strength in the muscles, and hallucinations. An unusual feature of narcolepsy is that it begins, rather than ends, with REM sleep, suggesting that it is probably linked to a fault in sleep-control centres. The disorder is rare, usually develops in late

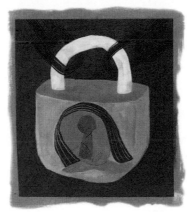

adolescence or early adulthood, and is largely hereditary (a narcoleptic's close relatives are sixty times more likely than other people to develop the disorder).

This innocent-sounding syndrome is extremely debilitating – not least because of the social implications of the susceptibility to falling asleep at any time. To make matters worse it is often many years before the condition is diagnosed. One of the most tell-tale signs is that strong emotions can bring on an attack, ranging from becoming overwhelmed by the action in a movie to (rather unromantically) falling asleep while making love.

Although conventional medicine usually recommends prescription drugs to combat narcolepsy, it can also be effectively tackled by napping. Sufferers should plan three or four naps throughout the day, each lasting approximately twenty minutes (but not more than thirty). You should awaken feeling altogether refreshed (although bear in mind that it will take a few minutes for full alertness to return), and the risk of untimely sleep should be greatly reduced. Keeping consistently to the regime of napping probably means that you will need to take naps at work (enlist the support of your colleagues to provide a suitable place for you), as well as, of course, napping at home.

Stepping Out of Time

Our biological clock and its proximity in the brain to the optic nerve help to synchronize our sleep with the daily cycle of light and dark. However, imagine how difficult life would be if the clock stepped out of time – if the usual 24-hour cycle by which the rest of the world lives became elusive to us and our body dictated its own sleep–wake agenda. There are a number of disorders, known as circadian disorders, in which the biological clock runs either on slow, fast or irregular. The three best-known are called *phase delay*, *phase advance* and *non-24-hour-sleep–wake syndrome*.

Phase delay affects mostly adolescents. Sufferers remain alert well into the early hours and then find it hard to wake up before midday. In stimulant-dependant societies, phase delay can lead to caffeine and nicotine dependency, as sufferers rely upon these two drugs to increase their alertness in the morning (when their biological clock thinks they should still be asleep). In the worst cases, alcohol dependency develops too because sufferers drink in order to be able to fall asleep. Unsurprisingly, all these factors lead to other health problems, and the sufferer's anxiety about lost sleep can lead to full-blown insomnia.

Phase advance is the opposite syndrome and occurs mainly in the elderly. Sleep can begin as early as between 6pm and 8pm and finish around 3am. And the non-24-hour-sleep–wake syndrome occurs when a person's biological clock runs continuously slowly so that for a time the sufferer is synchronized with the rest of society, but this synchronicity slips away.

All circadian disorders are best tackled using light: the exercise (opposite) suggests how this can help.

Exercise 18

SYNCHRONIZING CLOCKS

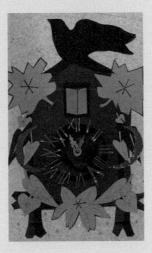

This exercise presents a complete action plan, including how to manipulate light, for sufferers of phase advance or phase delay syndrome. (Note: we all have a tendency to be a lark or owl – we have a circadian disorder only when this tendency is acute.)

1. Try to keep a constant routine. At weekends get up and go to bed at the same time as during the week. This should help to readjust your body clock.

2. Light during the evening can retard the biological clock to help those with phase advance syndrome – unfortunately, though, the light has to be very bright (see p.145). If you suffer from phase advance, avoid exposing yourself to daylight in the morning (even wearing sunglasses can help) and spend two hours in bright sunshine each afternoon. Hang heavy drapes or shades in your bedroom so that the dawn is masked, and shut the bedroom door to prevent light filtering in from other rooms.

3. If you suffer from phase delay, light in the early morning can help speed up the clock. It is also inadvisable to drink caffeine less than 10 hours before you go to bed. Although this may seem harsh – do not be tempted! Caffeine is a powerful drug that has longlasting effects and can seriously disrupt your sleep.

Crossing the World's Time Zones

If you have ever been on a long-haul journey, you will probably have experienced the frustrating effects of *jetlag* — especially irritating if arriving on a long-awaited vacation results in a day spent sleeping! Jetlag is the inability to sleep at the right time or being drowsy and sleepy at the wrong time, according to the time zone in which we find ourselves — quite literally, it is a mismatch between our biological clock and the clocks at our destination. As a general guide, the body takes roughly one day for each time zone travelled to adjust to the new cycle of day and night. With this in mind, most people can travel comfortably through three time zones without the need for specific counteractive measures (it is like going to sleep three hours later or earlier than normal).

Flying westwards, travelling backward in time, is more compatible with the biological clock than flying eastwards, because the body clock's natural cycle usually lasts slightly longer than a day. This tendency is encouraged by the time change, which lengthens the day. When we travel from West to East, the day shortens and this runs counter to the biological clock's natural drift, making it harder to adjust. Long-distance eastbound passengers suffer greater mental and physical problems which affect overall performance: baseball teams who fly eastwards for a game will, on average, reduce their score by as much as two runs!

Difficulties with jetlag can be cured using light. The best time to "reset" your body clock is at about 4am (departure point time). Exposure to bright light immediately before this time will delay your clock — helpful when going east — and exposure one to two hours after will advance it, aiding westward travel.

Exercise 19

DEALING WITH JETLAG

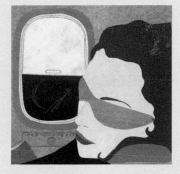

This exercise presents a complete strategy for coping with a long-distance flight, with the aim of minimizing the effects on your body clock so that you can enjoy your destination to the full.

1. The day before your flight, ensure that you eat three balanced meals, including at least five servings of fruit or green vegetables and one serving of a protein-rich food such as white fish or meat, or tofu.

2. During the flight set your watch to the local time at your destination. Note what extraordinary times the airline feeds you and try to keep back a roll or biscuit to eat at a "normal' mealtime according to the time at your destination.

3. Take an eye mask and ear plugs with you on the flight. Use the mask and your seat's "nightlight" to reflect the time at your destination — wear the mask if it is nighttime where you are going, and keep the light on and mask off if it is daytime.

4. Drink plenty of water throughout the flight. This will prevent dehydration and will also help to mobilize your energy reserves for your arrival. Avoid alcohol.

5. Take regular walks up and down the aisle. Try some simple stretching exercises in your seat: straighten your legs and point and flex your toes; or stretch your arms high above your head. Do both these exercises for one minute every two hours.

6. When you arrive at your destination, use your diet to help control your wakefulness: high-protein meals will increase your alertness and high-carbohydrate meals will make you feel more sleepy.

Working in Shifts

Studies of nurses have shown that the ones who cope best with shift work are those whose biological clock actually starts to adjust to the shift pattern. If a nurse works between the hours of midnight and 7am, the biological clock adjusts so that it recognizes the time when they get home as the beginning of a period of sleep, and when they wake up in the evening as the beginning of a period of wakefulness. Nurses who find shift work difficult seem to have biological clocks that are unadapted to the altered pattern of day and night — these nurses are representative of the problems faced by three-quarters of the world's shiftworkers.

Most importantly, we need to remember that the biological clock relies on light to regulate its time. With this in mind we should make sure that our environment is specially adapted to our lifestyle. Daylight must be prevented from setting the clock so that we cannot sleep during the day. In most

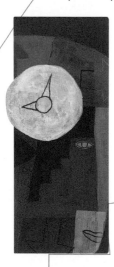

bedrooms light filters in through the drapes or shades because they are ill-fitting. If you work shifts make sure that your drapes keep out all light — and that means fastening the edges to the wall if necessary. Also, make sure that the door fits its frame perfectly — this will prevent light from filtering in from other rooms in the house when the door is closed. (Similarly, try to ensure that the sounds of the daytime are kept out of your bedroom. Fit your windows with double or even triple glazing and hang a heavy bedroom door.)

When a nightshift worker leaves work in the morning, almost certainly the light of dawn affects the biological clock, prompting it to adjust to 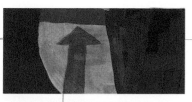 daytime. Specially adapted sunglasses are available which prevent the resetting — but they are unsuitable if you have to drive home.

To ensure high levels of alertness and vigilance in night-staff and in astronauts during space-shuttle missions, the space organization NASA uses bright 10,000-lux lights (home lighting produces only a few hundred lux) to reset its workforce's biological clocks. Other work-critical organizations, such as nuclear power stations, are beginning to do the same. After all, some of the worst environmental disasters over the last decades, including the accidents at Three Mile Island and Chernobyl and the grounding of the *Exxon Valdez*, occurred during the "zombie zone" (between 3am and 5am), when nightworkers are most sleepy.

ADJUSTING TO SHIFT WORK

Here is a summary of the golden rules on how to encourage your body clock to adjust to working shifts.

• Avoid using alcohol or over-the-counter medicines to make you sleepy
• Ensure that the drapes or shades in your bedroom do not let in any light
• Invest in double-glazing or buy a good pair of earplugs to eliminate noise disturbance • Manipulate your body clock using light • Do not forget to exercise — this is just as important for the wellbeing (waking and sleeping) of people who work shifts as for the rest of us.

Coping with Snoring and Apnea

Research indicates that more than a third of all adults snore. This curious disorder generates nearly 80 dB of sound (a level which some countries class as industrial noise pollution) and yet it does not wake up the snorer (usually male) – even though it might wake the people next door! But, snoring can still disrupt the sleep of the snorer, making them drowsy the next day and even more likely to be involved in road traffic accidents. Before we look at ways to deal with snoring and the more serious, related problem of *sleep apnea*, it is important to understand what happens when we snore and why the disorder develops.

When we are asleep, our airways are kept open by the throat muscles and the muscles that control the tongue and the soft palate (the tissues toward the back of the mouth). If these muscles are weak, the airways narrow and vibrate as we inhale, causing the sounds of snoring. There are many factors that increase the likelihood of snoring: aging (as we get older our mouth and throat muscles weaken), being overweight, smoking, consuming large amounts of alcohol, even sleeping on our back. Children are likely to snore if they have tonsilitis.

While for most people snoring may not constitute a health problem, sleep apnea is a much more serious condition. It occurs when the breathing passages of sufferers become temporarily obstructed as the tissues of the soft palate are sucked closed. This stops the person breathing. Their brain registers that no air is getting into the lungs and sends signals to the breathing muscles to try harder. The pause in breathing often ends with a loud snore as the obstructed airway is cleared, and the

Exercise 20

A SWANSONG FOR SNORES

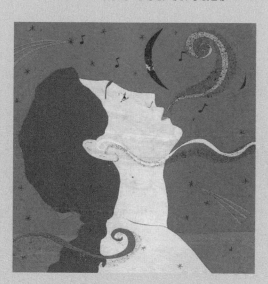

Dr Elizabeth Scott, a medical adviser to a Scottish orchestra, real-ized that professional singers rarely snore because of muscles they develop, so she devised a series of exercises to help non-singing snorers. Practise the following sitting comfortably in a chair.

1. Begin by strengthening the diaphragm. Breathe in, taking short, gasping breaths. Breathe out in a slow exhalation through pinched lips (as if playing a trumpet). As you reach the end of the breath, smile, so that the muscles at the back of the nose and upper throat tighten. Repeat for one minute, twice a day.

2. Look in the mirror and smile. Flare your nostrils and raise your eyebrows — as if in surprise. Relax your face. This strengthens the muscles in your face and at the back of your nose and upper throat. Repeat for one minute, twice a day.

3. Now try a singing exercise. Begin by singing the tune of a verse from a favourite song but, instead of singing the words, for each note sing the sound "ho". Then repeat the tune singing the sound "hee". Gradually increase the number of repetitions (alternating "ho" and "hee") until you are able to sing the song for three minutes in this way. Do this singing exercise once a day.

person wakes momentarily – for such a brief period that they are rarely aware of it. In severe cases the apneic may wake up aware that they cannot breathe, which can be very frightening. If the pause in breathing happens during REM sleep, when the body is virtually paralyzed, the lungs may take longer to respond to the brain's signals that it is receiving less oxygen, making the condition particularly dangerous. As interruptions to breathing can occur up to 300 times per night, the sufferers' sleep is severely disrupted and they experience very little deep or REM sleep. As a result of such unrefreshing sleep, sleep apneics can wake up feeling irritable, groggy and uncoordinated. They also often experience morning headaches. And if they try to make up for lost sleep by napping during the day, they often find this sleep unrefreshing too.

Apart from the serious dangers to a person's bodily health, one of the main consequences of sleep apnea is daytime sleepiness. The condition has been cited as a primary cause in the rise in road traffic accidents, with sufferers falling asleep unexpectedly at the wheel. It can also increase the apneic's risk of having a heart attack or a stroke – it is estimated that, in the USA, up to 3,000 people suffering from sleep apnea die from heart attacks every year. The life of asthmatics who are also apneic is gravely at risk during nighttime asthma attacks.

Most of the ways to reduce snoring also apply to sleep apnea. Neither condition can be treated reliably with drugs. Most treatments require the use of special mechanical devices. Self-help suggestions abound, and many are worth trying. To start, aim to improve your general breathing (the exercise on p.87 should help) and do the singing exercise on p.147, which offers a novel approach by exercising the muscles involved in breathing. You could also experiment with a nasal dilator – a device often used by athletes to improve their intake of oxygen. There are two types of nasal dilators: plastic clips, which are attached to the outside of the nose; and band-aid strips, which are placed across the nose. Nasal decongestants sometimes work, but take care not to use one that contains *ephedrine*, which disturbs sleep. In addition, do not use decongestants regularly as this will reduce their efficacy. It may sound strange, but if you have dentures, consider keeping them in overnight as they can help to prevent snoring, but discuss this first with your dentist. Take a good look at your lifestyle: try to exercise more and improve your diet; avoid alcohol within five hours of going to bed; and certainly do your best to stop smoking (see pp.80–81). Finally, to prevent you from lying flat on your back, try elevating the bed-head or use a specially-designed pillow that encourages you to sleep on your side.

Sufferers from severe sleep apnea may benefit from using a CPAP (continuous positive airway pressure) machine, which works by giving the user air at a slightly higher pressure than normal and thus keeps the airways open. It consists of a nasal mask, which is held in place by head straps. People who use CPAP machines often report a rapid and dramatic improvement in their sleep. There is also a surgical procedure called *uvulopalatoplasty*, which is used only in severe cases of sleep apnea. This drastic measure cauterizes the soft palate to stop it from closing and even vibrating (and so stops snoring); but if the surgery fails the apneic sometimes may no longer be able to use a CPAP machine because of the work done to the soft palate.

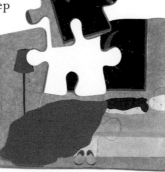

When Your Partner is the Problem

In a relationship all sleep disorders affect both partners. Insomniacs are restless even when they are trying not to disturb their bedfellow; hypersomniacs (people with excessive daytime sleepiness) invariably either suffer from a disturbance (such as loud snoring, sleep apnea or PLMS) or share a bed with someone who does; Restless Leg sufferers get up and walk to ease their strange sensations; and sleepwalkers get in and out of bed.

If your partner is disrupting your sleep, one of the most important things to remember is that they do not mean to! Their behaviour is not conscious and, invariably, if one partner's sleeping pattern is disrupting the other's, the results are distressing for both. So, although you may feel angry or frustrated, you should try to develop understanding and empathy and make a special effort to maintain the intimate connection that brought you together. The time spent in shared intimacy in the bed is one of the features of the most successful long-term relationships. If your partner is disrupting your sleep, make sure that the bed can

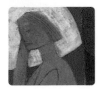

remain a place of pleasure — reinforce close contact by nurturing rich and pleasurable sexual activity.

Work together toward finding a solution to the sleep problems. Do everything you can to avoid separate rooms, but as your sleep deficits may build up, on the occasional weekend you could catch up by sleeping elsewhere. However, do not spend longer than usual in bed as this may disrupt your biological clock: remember the difference between short and long sleepers — short sleepers' sleep is

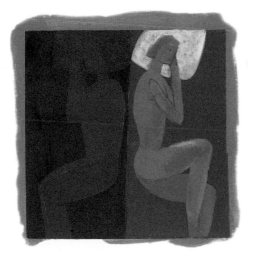

more intense, just like catch-up sleep. Do not panic over sleep loss – given a chance, sleep will look after itself.

If your partner suffers from PLMS or Restless Legs, devise an aromatherapy oil massage that you can give him or her before bed. This will relax the sufferer's legs, but it will also relax you too. If the problem is snoring or sleep apnea, try the singing exercise on p.147 together. Practising such exercises (even if you do not have the disorder for which they are intended) is positive action, and by tackling the problem together you offer a supportive hand to your partner and at the same time optimize the opportunity for your own sleep.

There is one disorder whose effects can be more difficult to tackle. In *REM behaviour disorder*, most commonly seen in men, the paralysis that usually accompanies dreaming sleep is absent, and dreams are acted out. This can be very frightening for partners, who are often physically as well as emotionally bruised by the disorder. This is one condition for which pharmacological treatment is desirable (and even this sometimes does not help). However, take heart – the condition is extremely rare.

Conclusion

Whatever our race, creed or culture, we all sleep. And people in all cultures suffer from sleep disorders. The universality of sleeping problems has led to the development of many therapies. It has been my aim in this book to give you all the basic information you need to improve the way you sleep – and hence I have explored many different approaches. And although, for example, Chinese and Indian systems of medicine are not readily compatible with Western science, I have included a wealth of techniques, from these and other sources, that can be drawn upon to help you improve your sleep.

However, if you are disappointed that you have not found a "magic" cure for your sleep problem, it is worth remembering that there are no quick-fixes. All ongoing therapies take time because the process of learning itself takes time. Be patient, and stick with your method long enough to give it a chance to work. If then you see no improvement, try another approach.

Sleep research is a relatively young science, having only really developed over the past fifty years. The more interest that can be generated in sleep science, the more knowledge about sleep and its disorders will become available to help us to improve our sleep. Perhaps in another fifty years, our understanding of sleep will have progressed by such leaps and bounds that sleep disorders will be a rarity! But in the meantime, remember that good sleep is the key to a long, healthy and fulfilling life. Don't give up until you attain it!

Bibliography

Ball, N. and N. Hough,
The Sleep Solution, Vermilion,
London, 1998; Ulysses Press,
Berkeley, 1998

Chopra, D.,
Restful Sleep, Rider/Ebury Press,
London, 1994; Crown
Publishing, New York, 1996

Craze, R.,
Feng Shui for Beginners, Hodder &
Stoughton, London, 1994;
Trafalgar Square, Vermont,
1999.

Dement, W. C. with C. Vaughan,
The Promise of Sleep, Macmillan,
London, 1999; Random House,
New York, 1999

Flaws, B.,
Curing Insomnia Naturally, Blue Poppy
Press, Boulder, Colorado, 1997.

Fontana, D.,
Learn to Meditate, Duncan Baird,
London, 1998; Chronicle Books,
San Francisco, 1999

George, M.,
Learn to Relax, Duncan Baird,
London, 1998; Chronicle Books,
San Francisco, 1997

Idzikowski, C.,
The Insomnia Kit, Newleaf, Dublin,
1999; Viking Penguin, New York,
1999

Lavery, S.,
The Healing Power of Sleep, Gaia
Books, London, 1997.

Mitchell, E. (ed.),
Your Body's Energy, Duncan
Baird/Mitchell Beazley, London,
1998; Macmillan Publishing,
New York 1998

Scott, E.,
The Natural Way to Stop Snoring,
Orion, London, 1995.

Shapiro, C.M. (ed.),
The ABC of Sleep Disorders, BMJ
Publications, London, 1993;
Login Brothers Book Company,
New York, 1994

Too, L.,
Essential Feng Shui, Rider/Ebury
Press, London, 1998; Ballantine
Books, New York, 1999

Van Straten, M.,
The Good Sleep Guide, Kyle Cathie,
London, 1996; Trafalgar Square,
Vermont, 1996

Index

A

acupressure 90, 91

adolescents 22, 140

adrenaline *see* epinephrine

affirmations 102–5

aggression 106

alcohol, sleep and 23, 63, 78, 79–80, 130, 149

alertness measurement 13, 37

alpha waves 34, 108

anger 106, 107

anxiety 23, 62, 102–5, 114, 116

  herbal medicine and 96

  insomnia and 128–9

apnea *see* sleep apnea

Aristotle 12, 27

aromatherapy 96–9, 151

Aserinsky, Eugene 13, 35

B

babies 60–63, 119

baths 92, 93, 96, 99, 121

bedding 57, 63

bedrooms 47, 130

  colour schemes 64

  Feng Shui and 66–9

  noise-free 118–19

  temperature 49

beds 32, 54–7

  position of 49, 68

  sharing 58–9, 60–63, 150

bedtime routines 36, 93, 120–121, 141

Berger, Hans 12–13, 34

beta waves 34

beverages, sleep and 78–80

biological clock 27, 29–31, 44–5, 50, 64, 101, 151

  jetlag and 142, 143

  shiftwork and 144–5

  sleep disorders and 140, 141

blinds *see* shades

Bodhidharma 89

body temperature 50, 57, 74, 92

  exercise and 84

Bootzin, Richard 129

Bootzin Stimulus Control 128, 129

Braid, James 116

brain, the

  bedtime and 36, 120

  behaviour during sleep 34–5

  biological clock 27, 30

  electrical activity 13, 27, 34, 42

  sleep and 12–15, 17, 32–3, 38, 52–3, 122–4

brain waves 34–5, 52–3, 108

breathing exercises 86, 87, 89, 148

C

caffeine 76, 78–9, 130, 140, 141
Californian Poppy 97
camomile 61
  Roman Camomile 99
children
  bedtime and 121
  sleeping arrangements for 63
  sleeping with 60–63
Chinese Horoscope 70, 71
cigarettes 78, 80–81
circadian disorders 140, 141
consciousness 33, 38
Corpse Pose (yoga) 86
CPAP (continuous positive
  airway pressure) machine 149
cramp *see* legs, nocturnal cramps in
curtains *see* drapes

D

decongestants 149
delta waves 35
dentures, snoring and 149
depression
  insomnia and 131
  lavender and 98
Descartes, René 33
drapes 51, 64, 141, 144
dream catchers 123
dream cues 124
dreaming sleep *see* REM sleep

dreams 17, 22, 34, 39, 43, 122–5
dreamless sleep 27, 42
  memory aid 42, 123
  recall of 124, 125
  see also hallucinations;
    nightmares; visions
drowsiness 15, 38, 44
duvets 57

E

Eaglewood incense 93
EEG (electroencephalogram) 13,
  34, 35, 42, 52
encephalitis lethargica 32
energy
  conservation, during sleep 16
  levels 46
environment, sleep and 30, 49–71
ephedrine 149
epinephrine
  anger and 106
  nicotine and 81
exercise (physical) 23, 82–5, 106,
  130, 149

F

Feng Shui 49, 66–71
fennel tea 61
fluids 76–7
food
  additives and sleep quality 76

effects on sleep 74–7
Freud, Sigmund 122, 124
futons 54, 57

G
Gattefosse, Henri 96

H
hallucinations 39, 138
  see also dreams; nightmares; visions
hammocks 54, 57
Hartmann, Ernest 123, 124
head position 68–9, 70, 71
herbal medicine 96–9
herbal teas 61, 79, 80, 99
Hinduism, consciousness and 42
hops 97–8
hormones 28, 41
horoscopes, Chinese 70, 71
humidity 51
hypnagogic dreams 34, 39
hypnopompia 39
hypnosis 81, 116–17

I
insomnia 46, 82, 90, 102–125,
  128–31, 140
  herbal medicine and 96–9
  hypnosis and 116–17
  see also sleeplessness
irritability 42, 47, 106

J
Jamaican Dogwood 98
jetlag 142–3
Jung, Carl 112, 122–3, 124

K
Kleitman, Nathaniel 13, 15, 35
Kua numbers 70, 71

L
Lady's Slipper 98
"larks" 31
lavender 96, 98
legs
  nocturnal cramps in
    (Charley-horse) 133
  Restless Legs 132–3, 150, 151
lifestyle
  sleep and 23, 46, 73, 82
  snoring and 149
light 47, 64, 140, 141
light and dark cycles 18
long sleepers 40

M
magnesium, sleep quality and 76
mammals, sleep behaviour in 18–19
massage
  before bed 58–9, 82–3
  pre-sleep face massage 95
  sleep and 94

mattresses 47, 49, 54–7, 63
  support mattresses 56
  water-filled 57
medicine, herbal 96–9
meditation 58, 88, 106, 108–115,
  124, 130
  candle-flame 109
  mandalas and yantras 112, 113
  stages of 110–11
  visual 112–13, 114–15
  see also relaxation; visualization
melatonin 28, 64
mental health 46–7
Mesmer, Franz Anton 116
metabolism 16, 19, 74–5, 84, 108
mind, sleep and 101–125
music, sleep preparation and 119

N
naps 20, 23, 45, 138, 148
narcolepsy 138–9
nasal devices, aids to sleep 149
nature, sleep behaviour in 12, 18–19
nicotine, sleep and 80–81
night terrors 135
nightcap recipe 74
nightmares 62, 135, 136–7
  cheese and 75
  see also dreams
nightwear 51
noise 47, 52–3, 118–19

O
opium poppy 97
"owls" 31

P
Pa Kua chart 69, 70, 71
paradoxical sleep see REM sleep
paralysis, sleep 16, 42–3, 138
partner, sharing bed with 58–9,
  150–151
peppermint 61, 99
Periodic Limb Movement Syndrome
  (PLMS) 133, 150–151
pillows 56, 97, 149
plants, sleep and 18
Plato 27
Polidori, Dr John 134
posture, sleeping 19, 56

Q
Qi 66–9, 88, 90

R
rapid eye movemment sleep
  see REM sleep
recall, of dreams 124, 125
relaxation 38, 108, 112, 130
  techniques 119, 120, 121
  see also meditation;
  visualization
REM behaviour disorder 151

REM sleep 13, 15, 27, 35, 36, 41,
    42–3, 44, 52, 79, 122
  depression and 131
  memory aid 42
  sleep apnea and 148
  sleep disorders and 138
rest 12, 14, 16–17
Restless Legs 132–3, 150, 151
restlessness 132
rhythms
  circadian 30
  infradian 28
  see also biological clock
rituals, bedtime 120–121
Roman Camomile 99

S
seasons, effects on sleep 28–9
semi-consciousness 24
shades (blinds) 64
sheng chi 70, 71
shift work 44–5, 144–5
short sleepers 40, 44
siestas 20, 23
silence, sleep and 118
singing 147, 151
sleep
  age and 22
  apnea 46, 136, 146–9
  behaviour in nature 12, 17, 18–19
  controls 32, 38

cycles 15, 36, 43–4
  debt 40, 44–5
  deep sleep 15–16, 22, 35, 36,
    40–41, 43, 44, 52, 79
  diet and 74–7
  disorders see sleep disorders
  disrupted 23, 44, 63, 96, 106,
    118, 133, 146, 148
  duration of 20–21
  environment for 30, 33, 46, 47,
    49–71, 118
  evolution and 16–17
  falling asleep 27, 36, 38–9, 46,
    114
  herbs and 96–9
  improvement of 30–31, 33, 36,
    38, 43, 46, 96–9, 102–124
  journal 24, 25, 46, 77, 130
  light sleep 15, 16, 23, 34, 36,
    38–9, 40, 43, 52, 108
  newborn children and 60–63
  paralysis during 138
  patterns 27, 29, 24, 32
  preparation for 120–121
  quality 22–3, 29, 33, 44, 46–7,
    50, 58, 69, 74–7
  relationships and 58–9, 150–151
  routines and 120–121
  stages 13, 15, 27, 34–43, 44
sleep disorders 46, 127–51
  relationships and 150–151

see also circadian disorders;
   insomnia; narcolepsy;
   nightmares; paralysis; Restless
   Legs; sleep, apnea; snoring
"sleep drunkenness" 41
sleep-state misperception 128,
   130
sleepiness, daytime 148
   see also narcolepsy
sleeping sickness 32
"sleeping table" (used in journal)
   24, 25, 46, 77, 130
sleeping tablets 99
sleeplessness 41, 82, 88, 102, 109,
   128
   dreams and 39, 136
   herbs and 96—9
   see also insomnia
sleepwalking 62, 134, 150
smoking, sleep and 80—81, 149
snoring 53, 150
   coping with 146—9
"Spinning Technique", nightmares
   and 137
Spock, Benjamin, *Baby and Child Care*
   60—61

T
T'ai Chi 88, 90, 91, 106
temperature, sleep and 50—51, 63
tension 82, 86, 94

theta waves 34
thirst 76—7
thought management 102—5
tiredness 34, 44, 146

U
uvulopalatoplasty 149

V
valerian 99
visions (hypnagogia) 38
   see also dreams; hallucinations;
   nightmares
visualization 106, 114—15, 130
   dreams and 124
   see also meditation; relaxation
vitamin B-complex 75—6

W
wakefulness 14, 32—3, 35, 38, 88,
   138
water beds 54, 57
water consumption 76—7, 79
wellbeing 43, 46—7, 77
worry see anxiety

Y
yantras 112, 113
yin and *yang* 66, 88
yoga 86—7, 106
yogis 86, 108